S.S.F. Public Library
West Orange
840 West Orange Ave.
South San Francisco, CA 94080

South San Francisco Public Library

3 9048 10920288 1

JUL 1 8

Homeless Youth
and the
Search for Stability

D1565171

S.S.F. Public Library
West Orange
840 West Orange Ave.
South San Francisco, CA 94080

Homeless Youth
and the
Search for Stability

JEFF KARABANOW

SEAN KIDD

TYLER FREDERICK

JEAN HUGHES

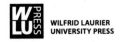

WILFRID LAURIER
UNIVERSITY PRESS

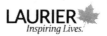

Wilfrid Laurier University Press acknowledges the support of the
Canada Council for the Arts for our publishing program. We acknowledge the
financial support of the Government of Canada through the Canada Book Fund for
our publishing activities. This work was supported by the Research Support Fund.

  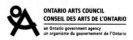

Library and Archives Canada Cataloguing in Publication

Karabanow, Jeff, 1969–, author
Homeless youth and the search for stability / Jeff Karabanow,
Sean Kidd, Tyler Frederick, Jean Hughes.

Includes bibliographical references and index.
Issued in print and electronic formats.
ISBN 978-1-77112-333-4 (softcover).—ISBN 978-1-77112-335-8 (EPUB).—
ISBN 978-1-77112-334-1 (PDF)

1. Homeless youth—Canada. 2. Homeless youth—Canada—Case studies.
I. Kidd, Sean, 1973–, author II. Frederick, Tyler, 1980–, author
III. Hughes, Jean, [date], author IV. Title.

HV4509.K373 2018   362.7'7569200971   C2017-905685-9
                                                     C2017-905686-7

Front-cover photo by Steve Douglas. Cover design by hwtstudio.com.
Interior design by Janette Thompson (Jansom).

© 2018 Wilfrid Laurier University Press
Waterloo, Ontario, Canada
www.wlupress.wlu.ca

This book is printed on FSC® certified paper and is certified Ecologo.
It contains post-consumer fibre, is processed chlorine free,
and is manufactured using biogas energy.

Printed in Canada

Every reasonable effort has been made to acquire permission for copyright material
used in this text, and to acknowledge all such indebtedness accurately. Any errors and
omissions called to the publisher's attention will be corrected in future printings.

No part of this publication may be reproduced, stored in a retrieval system,
or transmitted, in any form or by any means, without the prior written consent
of the publisher or a licence from the Canadian Copyright Licensing Agency
(Access Copyright). For an Access Copyright licence, visit
http://www.accesscopyright.ca or call toll free to 1-800-893-5777.

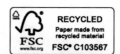

CONTENTS

CHAPTER 1

Introduction

This is a story about courage, fortitude, strength, adversity, and, at times, simply bad luck. It is a glimpse into the lives of young people who have lived on the street, and within this larger context, we explore a small segment of that population who have been able to leave street life, at least for the moment, and have secured some form of stable housing. Ultimately, this becomes a story of fragility, complexity, living "on the edge," and (re)-building identity.

The book is based on a Social Sciences and Humanities Research Council of Canada (SSHRC)-funded study conducted between 2011 and 2014, which took place in two Canadian cities: Halifax, a mid-size coastal city, and Toronto, Canada's largest and most diverse urban centre. Using a longitudinal mixed-method research approach (both in-depth qualitative interviews and questionnaires/scales), we interviewed former homeless youth (twenty-one from Nova Scotia and thirty from Toronto) over the course of one year, four separate times at three-month intervals. Fifty-one participants were recruited across the two sites, including twenty-seven females and twenty-four males, with a mean age of twenty-one years (range from seventeen to twenty-five); thirteen of the participants were mothers (nine in Halifax, and four in Toronto) (see Table 1 for more details about participants). This style of methodology provided us with a privileged entry into the lives of these young people for the year and allowed us to explore in more detail than cross-sectional analyses the complexities and nuances of street exiting over time. Few studies of street youth have been able to adopt a longitudinal stance, and even fewer have a mixed methodological foundation. Most research to date has focused on youth who are currently homeless, in a single urban centre, and has surveyed the youth at a single point in time to quantitatively capture

TABLE 1 Demographic characteristics of individuals studied (n = 51)

Variable	n (%)
Gender, male, n (%)	24 (47)
Age, mean years (standard deviation)	20.9 (2.2)
Percentage white, n (%)	24 (47)
Education, n (%)	
Less than high school	27 (53)
Completed high school	14 (27)
Attended trade/technical school	3 (6)
Completed trade/technical school	2 (4)
Attended university, not completed	4 (8)
Missing	1 (2)
Sexual orientation	
Heterosexual	29 (56)
Gay	5 (10)
Lesbian	2 (4)
Bisexual	9 (18)
Other	5 (10)
Missing	1 (2)
Children, n (% yes)	25 (49)
Employment status, n (%)	
Student	19 (37)
Employed part time/casual	8 (16)
Volunteer	3 (6)
Unemployed	21 (41)
Living situation time 1, n (%)	
Supportive housing, lives alone	6 (12)
Supportive housing, lives with others	18 (35)
Independent housing, lives alone	9 (18)
Independent housing, lives with others	13 (26)
Lives with parents in private dwelling	3 (6)
Missing	1 (2)
Months homeless	25.1 (27.5)
Months housed	8.8 (7.4)

risk factors. Other key facilitators of this inquiry include our experien-ces in the field and multidisciplinary lens (highlighted in Chapter 6), as well as arts-based participatory methods with work co-created with our research participants to support advocacy in this field (highlighted in Chapters 4 and 5).

Youth homelessness is a global problem affecting both high- and low-income countries (United Nations Educational, Scientific and Cultural Organization [UNESCO], 2014). Prevalence estimates for North America exceed one million in the United States (Kidd & Scrimenti, 2004; Perlman, Willard, Herbers, Cutuli, & Eyrich Garg, 2014) and forty thousand in Canada (Gaetz, Donaldson, Richter, & Gulliver, 2013). We define "homeless" or "street" youth as young people who do not have a permanent place to call home. They spend a significant amount of time on the street, in squats (usually abandoned buildings), and at shelters and support centres. Canadian research shows that the street youth popula-tion is diverse, complex, and heterogeneous, and encompasses a num-ber of subcultures, including hard-core street-entrenched young people, youth in and/or out of group homes and foster care, refugees and immi-grants, and young single mothers (Gaetz, O'Grady, Buccieri, Karabanow, & Marsolais, 2013; Coward Bucher, 2008; Karabanow, 2004a, 2008).

Relative to the large body of work examining pathways into youth homelessness and the risks associated with living on the streets, a limited amount of research has concentrated on pathways *out* of homelessness. Our study was designed to address this gap through in-depth, longitud-inal, mixed-methods examination of young people as they tried to transi-tion away from homelessness.

Why and how youth engage with street life is well documented. The causes and consequences of youth homelessness include family dysfunc-tion, abuse and trauma, exploitation, alienation, poverty, addiction, men-tal and physical illness, and service sector inadequacies (Edidin, Ganim, Hunter, & Karnik, 2012; Hagan & McCarthy, 1997; Hughes et al., 2010; Karabanow, 2004a, 2006, 2008; Kidd, 2004, 2006, 2013; Martijn & Sharpe 2006). Street cultures present complex and often dichotomous narratives: they can be sites of excitement, belonging, and acceptance, as well as exploitation, violence, and stress (Auerswald & Eyre 2002; Karabanow

2003, 2006; Karabanow et al., 2007). To survive in this context, youth engage in numerous activities, including trying to find work, asking for money from family and friends, panhandling, prostitution, survival sex (sex for food, shelter, etc.), drug dealing, and theft (Hagan & McCarthy, 1997; Karabanow, Hughes, Ticknor, Kidd, & Patterson, 2010). Once youth are on the streets, threats to physical and mental health are great, as demonstrated by extremely high morbidity and mortality rates in large part due to suicide and drug overdose (Roy et al. 2004; Roy, Haley, Boudreau, Leclerc, & Boivin, 2009).

The difficulty of surviving on the streets is clear from the large number of homeless youth who regularly lack shelter and go hungry, fall victim to physical and sexual assaults, abuse drugs and alcohol, and suffer from poor mental and physical health (Frederick, Chwalek, Hughes, Karabanow, & Kidd, 2014; Hughes et al., 2010; Karabanow et al., 2007; Kidd, 2004). Street life also carries significant social stigma. Most homeless youth regularly experience acrimonious interactions with the general public stemming from their appearance, survival techniques, and homeless (living in public space) status. This stigmatization leads to victimization and criminalization, and causes difficulty in finding work and housing (Karabanow, 2004a; Karabanow, Hughes, Ticknor, Kidd, & Patterson, 2009; Karabanow et al., 2010; Kidd, 2003, 2004; McKenzie-Mohr, Coates, & McLeod, 2012).

The topics of resilience, strength, hope, and survival have gained increasing attention in the North American literature on youth homelessness (Hughes et al., 2010; Karabanow, 2003, 2004a, 2004b, 2008; Kidd, 2003; Rew & Horner, 2003). There is also an emerging body of work that addresses the deeper cultural frameworks and senses of identity that determine how homeless youth understand and experience their world, and that define and drive their coping efforts (Karabanow, 2006). Garret et al. (2008) found that youth who successfully transition off the street demonstrate autonomy, self-reliance, and mainstream values, and develop relationships with other people who are off the street. Kidd and Davidson (2007) highlight the manner in which coping efforts were framed within youth's testing, adopting, and rejecting the various identities and self-concepts available in the street context. Youth who do not take on street value systems and norms find it more difficult to survive on the street, and they show much more motivation to use existing services. In contrast, youth who become part of street subcultures and take on their value systems might experience a better quality of life in the street context, but they face far greater risks and are more difficult to engage in interventions (e.g., youth for whom sex-trade work has become the norm).

Although not focused specifically on exiting the streets, some longitudinal, quantitative studies have provided insight into this process, while considering the amount of time spent on and off the streets (Barber, Fonagy, Fultz, Simulinas, & Yates, 2005; Milburn et al., 2009; Rosenthal et al., 2007; Roy et al., 2014; Slesnick, Bartle-Haring, Dashora, Kang, & Aukward, 2008; Slesnick, Dashora, Letcher, Erdem, & Serovich, 2009; Tevendale, Comulada, & Lightfoot, 2011). The most consistent finding is that drug and alcohol abuse reduced the number of days housed (Rosenthal et al., 2007; Roy et al., 2014; Slesnick et al., 2008; Tevendale et al., 2011). Number of days housed was linked positively with having connections with peers and family (Milburn et al., 2009; Slesnick et al., 2009), demonstrating less risk behaviour (Slesnick et al., 2008), being female (Slesnick et al., 2008), having past and current educational experience (Milburn et al., 2009; Roy et al., 2014), being younger, and having been homeless for a shorter period of time (Tevendale et al., 2011). Somewhat less intuitive are findings that youth who had left home involuntarily (i.e., "throwaways") were more likely to find housing (Tevendale et al., 2011), as were youth experiencing mental health problems (Roy et al., 2014). Interpretations of these findings suggest that pathways off the streets can depend on self-concept. For example, emotional distress might indicate youth who feel that they do not belong, or fit in, on the streets and therefore possess greater motivation to find housing.

Canadian studies by Karabanow and colleagues (Karabanow, 2006, 2008; Karabanow, Clement, Carson, & Crane, 2005) involved some preliminary exploration into trajectories leading away from street life. These cross-sectional studies explored how Canadian street youth successfully and unsuccessfully disengaged from street culture over the short term in six Canadian cities. The resulting data identified barriers to successful transitions, including addictions, trauma, discrimination, unemployment, and breaking ties with street culture and street friends (Karabanow, 2008; Karabanow et al., 2010).

In contrast to the descriptive literature, very little formal research is available regarding interventions with this population, and what exists is primarily focused upon individual factors. This is likely due in part to the complex nature of the needs and relevant interventions for homeless youth, which are often highly individualized, multi-component, and long term. This greatly limits the application of trial designs with the resources typically available for such research. More importantly, the instability inherent to this population makes engagement difficulties and attrition major problems in study design and logistics. A range of policy solutions have been generated in Canada, though the data that might speak to their effectiveness are lacking. Criminalization is a common response, most notably the "Safe Streets" acts implemented in many jurisdictions in the past twenty years (Quirouette, Frederick, Hughes, Karabanow, & Kidd, 2016). Other key domains that, arguably, have not been comprehensively addressed include issues such as jail diversion, supports available to youth who age out of child protection services, mental health supports for children and families available through the education system, and the disconnect between child and adult services (Kidd & Davidson, 2007). Funding in this sector is highly complex and competitive, and systematic, sustained approaches are lacking—leaving most organizations underfunded and burdened with the management of income through combinations of philanthropy, short-term grants from three levels of government, and inconsistent transfers of funds. There are, however, exceptions: some cities are taking a sustained and systematic approach informed by evidence, as has been the case with housing first initiatives in Canada and elsewhere (Gaetz, Scott, & Gulliver, 2013).

At a service level, the overwhelming majority of services available are crisis oriented, taking the form of drop-ins and shelters. Constantly challenged at a resource level and applying a wide range of service models, these services lack clear research speaking to their effectiveness beyond counting the numbers of youth who engage (Slesnick et al., 2009). It is clear, however, that interventions need to be tailored specifically to a youth population and the diversity therein—if minimally evidenced by observations such as less impact for this population through intensive case management (Altena, Brilleslijper, & Wolf, 2010; Slesnick et al., 2009) and a more challenging context for implementing housing first

(Kozloff et al., 2016). In terms of specific interventions, modest bodies of work have emerged suggesting effective approaches in areas of HIV and sexual health, ecologically based family therapy, motivational interventions for substance use, and the community reinforcement model of cognitive behavioural therapy for mental health challenges (Baer, Peterson, & Wells, 2004; Kidd, 2003; Peterson, Baer, Wells, Ginzler, & Garrett, 2006; Slesnick & Prestopnik, 2005; Slesnick et al., 2009; Slesnick, Prestopnik, Meyers, & Glassman, 2007).

Given the overall lack of population-level data, whether descriptive or in the form of representative intervention studies, it is very difficult to unpack what considerations might be unique to Canada versus other high-income countries. There are clear commonalities across contexts, with similar reports and rates of childhood adversity, street victimization, mental health and addiction challenges, and the service structures and policies that have been designed to address these issues. While difficult to compare with populations in other countries, the recently released National Homeless Youth Survey has provided a unique source of information about homeless youth (Gaetz, O'Grady, Kidd, & Schwan, 2016). This survey reinforced observations of the high degree of diversity among youth accessing homeless-oriented services. Key specific considerations included the far greater adversity faced by lesbian, gay, bisexual, queer, and two-spirited (LGBQ2S) youth, differing profiles of risk as a function of racialized and Indigenous identity, and greater adversity faced by female youth.

Along with the paucity of information available about interventions, a critical and understudied area involves the transition process out of homelessness for youth. This gap is highly apparent among service providers and is evident in a body of research that focuses almost exclusively on street adversity. We do not have a good understanding of the ways in which young people transition away from being homeless once they are housed, and how these dynamics influence their sense of self and the building/rebuilding of their identity and place in their community. This book explicitly takes up the question of how we can better understand the lived experiences of young people once they have left street life. In the simplest of terms, these chapters, while diverse, concern themselves with the question, asked by so many over the years, of what happens when youth leave the streets.

The importance and originality of this research project are significant. The financial and social costs of youth homelessness are high. Homeless youth suffer from poor physical and mental health (Hughes et al., 2010; Karabanow et al., 2007; Kidd, 2004). More than half spend time in jail: 62 percent in 2003, up from 56 percent in 1999 according to the Public Health Agency of Canada (2006). They have extremely high mortality rates (Roy et al., 2004; Shaw & Dorling, 1998) and are a visible urban reminder of shortcomings in our institutions, services, and supports. It costs approximately $30,000 to $40,000 each year to house a young person in the shelter system and $100,000 a year to house a youth in detention (Evenson & Barr, 2009). The growing number of homeless youth, coupled with the costs of "warehousing" them (rather than responding to their complex needs during a critical developmental stage), indicates the vital importance of understanding how youth can be successful in street exiting. It is essential to understand the factors that impede or facilitate exiting the streets in order to develop effective interventions, supports, and policies.

Accordingly, the primary goal of this book is to relate the lived experiences of homeless youth as they negotiate the individual, socio-cultural, and economic tensions of transitioning out of homelessness and street contexts and cultures. We tackle this inquiry through a variety of complementary lenses.

Chapter 2 takes up an exploration of the lives of formerly homeless young people as they begin their journey towards housing stability, using qualitative analyses to shed light on how youth exit the street. This chapter speaks to how youth *actually* navigate pathways out of homelessness to find and maintain housing and a sense of stability, and the trajectories that shape these pathways. At a broad level we see the transition away from homelessness as a four-stage process that youth move through in a series of cycles and spirals as they experience setbacks and encounter obstacles. We have identified a series of key factors relevant to each stage in this broad transition. In this way we can conceptualize the transition from homelessness as a series of trajectories along these factors. Conceptualizing the transition from homelessness in this way is valuable because it recognizes the many factors and components that underlie such a significant transition, as well as the diversity and complexity that characterize homeless young people and their pathways out of homelessness.

It also acknowledges that the transition from homelessness is not separate from the pathways that we all travel as we struggle to realize our goals and establish happy and fulfilling lives.

Chapter 3 launches from the previous conceptual discussion to focus on case studies that showcase the efforts of young people to sustain stability after a lengthy period of homelessness. We use case studies to examine the narratives of four participants in order to illustrate key stages of this process and provide critical insights into the complexity of pathways in and out of stability for youth.

The fourth chapter is an intentional challenge to typical research processes and putting those reflexive concerns into practice. Framing youth homelessness as a "wicked" social problem, in this chapter we attempt to push past the typical frustration with how to end a research project, typically confined to knowledge dissemination activities. There is a consistent failure to generate research that can be translated into real-world impacts by transforming knowledge into action. In this chapter we describe a participatory process where participants and artists were engaged to communicate our research findings in comic book format. We argue that art can be used to tell stories and actively build critical narrative spaces that were either latent, or nonexistent, before acts of collective storytelling infused them with life. This sort of knowledge translation process pushes the envelope methodologically, as the participants and artists contribute to the researchers' agenda, forcing researchers to loosen control over the analytical agenda of the research process.

Chapter 5 presents a comic book narrative that was produced using the methods described in Chapter 4 and showcases some of the common substantive themes to have emerged throughout the study.

Chapter 6 examines how longitudinal research with street youth presents a set of messy ethical and methodological challenges for researchers. These challenges, which include grappling with field issues such as intervention, relationships, reciprocity, and risk, stretch the boundaries and limits of the formal research constructs that typically guide an ethnographic research undertaking. In this chapter we playfully, yet earnestly, explore epistemological questions based on the practical field research experiences of a team of both junior and senior researchers. We argue that researchers must be transparent and accountable in reporting how we collect data in the field with vulnerable youth populations, at the same time that we ask to what extent it is possible to explicitly, and accurately, acknowledge the inherent messiness of working with such populations. In this way, the chapter reflects on the actual research process, and it also presents questions and answers to help guide others conducting research with vulnerable populations such as street youth.

We hope this collection of chapters will contribute to an emerging literature about exiting homelessness, which is beginning to inform housing policy and practices nationally and internationally. This book as a whole is intended to extend this conversation, providing new ways to understand the conditions and contexts prerequisite to successful street exiting (see Chapters 2 and 3). At the same time, we somewhat mischievously point to the gaps and pretensions inherent in conducting research with vulnerable populations, while trying to envision research strategies and orientations that honour multiple ways of knowing and do not end with frustration or cynicism (see Chapters 4, 5, and 6). Our ultimate goals are to co-create knowledge with research participants and emphasize reflexivity in the research process, while still contributing empirical evidence to a scholarly body of literature.

We believe that this book will be of interest to multiple stakeholders. First and foremost, we developed the text for researchers to assist in building—both adding to and reinforcing—the existing knowledge base of homeless young people and their trajectories over a period of one year. We believe the book will also be useful to scholars and students interested in research design, contexts, and issues as they pertain to marginalized, impoverished youth populations. We also believe the book will be useful to service providers and policy-makers. In particular, we believe that the qualitative analyses and artwork will help build greater understanding of the ways in which service providers and policy-makers can make specific changes in how they are trained and work to ensure that positive, strengths-based approaches are employed in regulations and practice to ensure that homeless young people do not continue to be marginalized/ignored. Our approach was purposely designed in a way to address critical elements of interest to service providers (e.g., the importance of client-centred training for service providers), and policy-makers (e.g., the importance of inter-sectoral approaches to policy-related programing).

CHAPTER 2

Street-Exiting Framework

This chapter begins the examination of street-exiting processes and trajectories that youth experienced as they began the complex transition into "stable housing." This work is drawn from repeated conversations over a period of one year with fifty-one youth in Halifax, Nova Scotia, and Toronto, Ontario, all having recently made a move from outright homelessness to some form of stable housing. This chapter presents the qualitative findings of the thematic analysis of those narratives. The thematic framework will be followed, in Chapter 3, with a lens on stages of the exiting trajectories as illustrated by specific case examples.

METHOD

As noted in the introduction, the study was conducted between 2011 and 2014 in two Canadian urban settings; Halifax, a mid-size coastal city, and Toronto, Canada's largest and most diverse urban centre. Aside from being a much larger city and having relatively more ethnic diversity than Halifax, Toronto is characterized by a youth homelessness service sector that is larger—both in the number of services offered and the size of any given service. Both cities, for their geographic area, tend to be centres towards which youth from smaller and more rural areas gravitate in order to access supports, to find income, and to get away from pre-street contexts. Recruitment involved two phases, with one being referrals from local service providers and the second phase involving snowball sampling from the social networks of participants.

We sought youth between the ages of sixteen and twenty-five who reported a history of at least six months of past homelessness and who met the following criteria for stability:

- During the period since homelessness (two months to two years), housing had been steadily maintained with no substantial periods of homelessness (more than a few days) in the interim.
- Housing did not include shelters, prison, or temporarily staying with others (i.e., couch surfing).
- The individual was subjectively understood not to be at a significant risk of immediate homelessness (e.g., in the process of eviction).

A total of four interviews per participant took place over the course of one year, at four-month intervals. Descriptive information (age, gender, ethnicity, education, employment, housing history, street history) was assessed from single items in the baseline interview. Quantitative and qualitative data were collected at each of these time points. This chapter explores the qualitative findings.

Qualitative data were gathered through in-depth interview techniques (Johnson, 2002; Miller & Crabtree, 2004) with a modified life review approach (Clausen, 1998). In-depth interviews were used to gather detailed information (Miller & Crabtree, 2004, p. 189), and a life review provided information on past experiences and events, but also on meaning making and lived experience (Clausen, 1998). Particular attention was given to the process of exiting homelessness, including discussion of turning points, supports and barriers in the exiting process, and the impact that transitioning had on a participant's relationships, identity, emotions, life satisfaction, and physical and mental health. Interviews were guided by an open-ended interview schedule, but were conversational and exploratory in nature and ranged from forty-five minutes to three hours in length. The first interview focused on obtaining a life history that included a discussion of pre-homeless experiences and pathways onto and off the streets. Subsequent interviews focused on activities and experiences in the preceding four-month period and provided opportunities to elaborate upon, and further explore, emerging themes. All the interviews were audio-recorded and transcribed verbatim.

The purpose of the qualitative analysis was to employ "thick" qualitative interview data to identify the factors and processes shaping the housing stability of young people transitioning away from homelessness. Our analysis of the data was informed by Clausen's (1998) life review approach, which conceptualizes an individual's life history in terms of turning points and trajectories through roles and identities. We began by identifying the main turning points and life events as they related to housing stability on a case-by-case basis for the young people in our sample. We did so as a team by organizing their transcript data into trajectories (similar to Clausen's use of life charts) and then identifying the most prominent types of trajectories, stages within trajectories, and their determinants as articulated through the youths' narratives. Thematic analysis (articulating key themes that were enacted in the identified trajectories) followed Boyatzis' (1998) techniques for qualitative coding and theme development. Each of the Halifax and Toronto teams engaged in thematic analysis, coming together frequently as a group to review transcripts, develop codes, and cycle between theme development and their framing in trajectories, and bringing questions about themes back to participants for further elaboration in subsequent interviews.

Recruitment was split evenly between the two geographical locations. We tailored our recruitment to produce a diverse sample and to maintain a maximum degree of balance geographically and within sites. Participants were paid forty dollars for each of the four interviews and were provided with transit tokens. Interviews were conducted by graduate and undergraduate research assistants familiar with this population and associated service contexts.

CONTEXTUALIZING OUR FINDINGS

As described in Chapter 1, it was the complicated trajectory from the street to stable housing that sparked our curiosity, and this analysis speaks to the often complex and nuanced pathways experienced by our participants. Our youth participants had diverse experiences with their families, living on the streets, and interacting with formal and informal service providers. This diversity continued as participants worked through the process of finding accommodation perceived to be stable, and then attempted to distance themselves from street culture and build ties to mainstream environments. At the same time, the richness and depth of our longitudinal data have enabled us to identify discernable patterns in the exiting process that could prove valuable in the design of intervention strategies to assist youth as they exit the street. As we demonstrate in this chapter, the exiting process, in its most discernable sense, can be mapped out as a broad four-stage process: (1) turning point, (2) housing, (3) acceptance, and (4) achievement.

Given that the research was taking place in two unique settings, Halifax and Toronto, it is worth providing a quick note on the two sites. Although we were on the lookout for differences between the two locales, the reality is that there was significantly more similarity than difference. There were a few site-specific influences—for example, a transit strike in Halifax during the study period created significant barriers for many of the young people there, and Halifax has a smaller service sector—but overall the two groups of youth appeared to share many of the same struggles and processes in their pathway off the street. We feel that this similarity is actually worth emphasizing in that it speaks to the universality and systemic nature of the challenges faced by these young people. As the discussion below will illustrate, issues around a lack of affordable housing; the barriers created by criminal records; the challenges of exiting the Children's Aid system; the stigma of youth, homelessness, and poverty; and barriers to mental health care are shared across communities in Canada. Other challenges faced by the young people in our sample were similarly crosscutting as they reflected the unique challenges faced by youth as a group (particularly marginalized youth), including the challenges of figuring who they are and where they fit in the world, maturing, negotiating the complexity of peer and family relationships, and managing the lifelong impact of trauma.

Several significant dimensions shape our understanding of these trajectories for our sample as a whole. First and foremost, our participants must be seen as citizens rather than street kids. Much of our earlier work in this field has highlighted the pathology and stigmatization imputed in this characterization, as well as the fact that young people rarely refer to themselves in this way. As a young person in an earlier study (Karabanow, 1999) noted quite eloquently, "When I am out there [on the street] I'm a street kid ... when I'm here [at a particular youth shelter], I'm a human being" (p. 324).

At the same time, it is important to acknowledge that these youth depart from what youth study theorists would term "typical pathways" for emerging adulthood in which youth become more independent and explore various life possibilities for the future (Arnett, Žukauskienė, & Sugimura, 2014). As is evident in our case studies (Chapter 3), the youth in our study did not have the luxury of being able to dream about their future possibilities. Instead, their family situations—involving violence, neglect, poverty, and social isolation—forced them to live in the moment and to make spontaneous decisions to escape the trauma. Such decisions often resulted in the only alternative—homelessness and coping strategies involving drug misuse and mental health ruptures that put dreaming about the future, and any dreams of identity, on hold.

Sadly, there is growing evidence that traumatic events, such as abuse, neglect, severe deprivation, and exposure to violence, take a costly toll (Simpson, 2008). Youth with a history of trauma are vulnerable to getting stuck developmentally, or to growing more slowly and/or unevenly than one would otherwise. In addition, evidence also points to the serious impact of chronic substance abuse on youth development. Research is demonstrating ways in which alcohol and other drugs affect the growing brain, causing damage that may or may not be possible to repair (Simpson, 2008).

Ensconced within such atypical pathways, the youth we encountered, as others have found (Wenzel et al., 2012), experienced a sense of alienation, marginalization, exploitation, and victimization, amid pathways that are far more institutionally mitigated than their mainstream counterparts. Lacking support and care from adults, being abused and exploited, living in poor and disadvantaged environments, and being let down from both personal (family, friends) and systemic (school, child welfare, social assistance) structures of care, for these youth a compounding or amplification effect that tends to characterize their pathways. This amplification effect is striking insofar as it appears that many of these youth simply have "bad luck"; however, underpinning this luck is a tangle of personal and institutional factors that shape the daily experiences of these youth.

A second dimension that significantly contextualizes our understanding of these young people is the fact that they are indeed the success stories of the homeless population. In fact, their success is the compelling feature of this chapter, since our aim here is to explore the features of that success: How is it that these youth were able to exit street life and seemingly embrace what most of us would recognize as somewhat mainstream personal and institutional values and systems?

Simultaneously, however, the success of these youth is coloured by a fragility that characterizes both their personal selves and their institutional identities. Indeed, one of the core themes of the book (characterized poignantly in the comic book) is that the majority of these young people remain in a fragile state throughout their transitions to "non-street" life. This fragility has much to do with their *in-between* status. Not certain they have indeed been removed from street life, and by no means comfortable or accepted within mainstream civil society, these young people struggle with their sense of self—of who they are, what they desire, where they are going, and what they need. Given that for most youth living on the street, their memories of home were filled with trauma and upheaval, it is not surprising that while they would *dream* of leaving the streets and living in a stable environment, they were not sure how *to do it*. Indeed, one participant noted that she did not know where she "fit in," sagely describing the deep tensions that exist when dis-embedding oneself from street life and culture: "Everyone else is just telling me how good I'm doing and I don't know if I'm actually doing good or if it just looks more socially acceptable. Like I can't tell if I'm actually doing good or people just think I'm doing good because, like, it's easy, nicer on paper."

In addition, while the existential questions involving identity are endemic to mainstream youth as they move from adolescence to young adulthood, the queries become amplified when the consequences of not being able to sort them out are far more dire. Indeed, many youth find themselves back on the streets, or in detox, or forced to live in a shelter, but some seem to have a better chance than others. More specifically, a recent Canadian study has found that young people (eighteen to twenty-five years) who had a high-school degree, had a *formal* sector activity, and who had sought psychological help were more likely to reach residential stability, while being a man, injecting substances, and having an *informal* sector activity were associated with a decreased probability of reaching residential stability (Roy et al., 2016). Roy and colleagues (2016) argue that exposure to factors related to opportunities that promote social integration seem to increase one's chances of reaching residential stability, while factors related to high-level street entrenchment seem to interfere with stabilization.

A third contextual element is that these youth experience their worlds as highly stressed, strained, overwhelmed, and fragile, *even within the context of being stably housed*—another key theme to the comic book narrative. While being perceived by service providers and the general public as less at risk now that they are no longer labelled "street kids," for these youth new layers of risk emerge within their new environments that also result in feeling fragile. Participants shared stories of continued struggles and conflicts in their families, group home settings, youth shelters, and independent housing environments. Within these pathways, there were common themes of abuse or neglect, deep tensions with family members, feelings of marginalization, and ongoing struggles with mental health and/or harmful use of drugs and alcohol. Not surprising, as Mackelprang and colleagues (2014) have found, traumas perpetrated by a caregiver or close other are more detrimental to mental health functioning than those experiences in which the victim is not affiliated closely with the perpetrator. For a number of our study participants, their move from the streets to stable housing away from family did not resolve, nor end, family trauma.

Finally in this chapter, as we discuss the process of transitioning from homelessness, we focus on the movement from homelessness to mainstream social and economic inclusion. Although this transition is associated with many positive changes, we do not want to argue that this is solely a transition from bad to good, or negative to positive. Mainstream social and economic goals are not without their drawbacks. They are normative and foreclose the possibility of equally fulfilling alternatives. Mainstream social and economic inclusion is also not equally available to everyone given the structural constraints of our society. The pressure towards mainstream definitions of success and worth is particularly problematic for young people who must manage serious physical or mental disabilities in the absence of adequate societal supports.

THE PROCESS OF TRANSITIONING FROM HOMELESSNESS

At a broad level, this chapter sketches a four-stage process vis-à-vis transition away from homelessness. These stages emerged across the year of interviews with participants as they reflected on their past and current circumstances. The reality was that a year was not nearly long enough to capture the full process of transition for those who succeeded, or to map out the full cycle of repeated missed attempts and resolution through chronic homelessness into adulthood or death—a very real threat for many (Roy et al., 2014).

In addition, by no means is this a linear, unidirectional path. Rather, youth move through these stages in a series of cycles and spirals as they experience setbacks and encounter obstacles. Within each stage of the broad transition is a series of key factors (e.g., orientation, resources) that are relevant to that stage. We conceptualize the transition from homelessness as a series of trajectories along these factors. One's movement along the individual factors is connected to the broader transition, but the two are not perfectly correlated. Conceptualizing the transition from homelessness in this way is valuable because it recognizes the many factors and components that underlie such a significant transition, as well as the diversity and complexity that characterize homeless young people and their pathways out of homelessness.

Turning Points

The first stage in the transition away from homelessness is characterized by recognizable turning points: events or circumstances that prompt a young person to commit to active pursuit of housing stability. As illustrated in the interview passages below, specific turning points vary but can involve the following: receiving encouragement and support from family or a romantic partner (primarily in terms of a place to stay off the street, as a break from sleeping rough); experiencing a traumatic event that highlights the risks in their lives (such as a violent encounter, incarceration, or drug/alcohol overdose); simply getting sick and tired of the often mundane harshness of street survival; and, in some cases, experiencing a life-changing event, such as discovering that they are pregnant (for a deeper analysis of these dimensions, see Karabanow et al., 2010).

> I helped myself. This time when I got out of jail, I'm the only reason that I am where I am right now. I helped myself, I'm saying. And nobody can help you. Unless you really want it, you know? And the last couple times I completed [detox], I didn't change shit, you know? They weren't forcing me to either. It's just, I don't know. I just got tired of it, as I said. I got tired of the bullshit and I decided to change right for myself, you know?
>
> And it was really hard but it was basically I can either choose ice [crystal meth] or I can choose a boyfriend in my life that actually cares about me. So I basically didn't have a choice—I had to do it. And I am happy I quit drugs.

This initial stage tends to be a place of personal reflection for youth—to assess where they are and where they want to be in the near future. It may not be the first time that they are questioning their street status, but there is some dimension in this phase (possibly a "growing up" or "maturing" dynamic, as some participants explain) that allows them to consider a different existence. Finding purpose and aspects of a new identity are born here: glimpses of what it would be like to be off the street, having a place to call home, returning to school, and having non-street friends. And these glimpses begin to make their mark on the youth's sense of self. It is this first glimmer that propels youth to continue on the trajectory towards some form of non-street stability. These glimpses also reflect further brain development within the prefrontal cortex, resulting in enhanced thinking and emotional regulation—critical components of emotional intelligence (Goleman, 2006). Emotional intelligence involves self-awareness, self-management (self-control), social awareness, and interpersonal skills that enable one to (1) perceive emotions in oneself and others accurately; (2) use emotions to facilitate thinking; (3) understand emotions, emotional language, and the signals conveyed by emotions; and (4) manage/regulate emotions so as to attain specific goals (Mayer & Salovey, 1997). Emotional intelligence is highly important for building the prefrontal cortex—an area of the brain that continues to develop into the mid-twenties and helps reasoning, inhibition, planning, problem solving, decision making, and working memory (Goleman, 2006). Hence, youth in our study who were able to persevere with their intentions made a critical step forward in their overall development.

One of the key ingredients for this stage is having some form of support within the reflection phase: having someone to talk to, to lay out options and choices, to walk with them through varying routes, and to be there to provide comfort and care. At this stage, our participants tend to gain their support from social service workers rather than friends or family. At this early point, youth shelter workers, outreach workers, social workers, and/or housing workers tend to be the main players supporting and accompanying the youth in their search for housing options. Indeed, formal supports are often key in providing services (counselling, housing, education, employment) and assisting street youth in finding a voice, sense of purpose, positive self-identity, and social and self-awareness (Farrar, Schwartz, & Austin, 2011; Karabanow, 2004a, 2004b; Rodrigues Coser et al., 2014). In many ways this process is aligned with the Canadian-wide movement towards housing first principles: get people housed, and then provide consumer-driven supports ("Housing First Principles," 2017).

Housing

The second broad stage involves youth acquiring the basic features of stability, housing being the most fundamental. Other studies have shown similar results; indeed, not having stable housing has been found to be the most important factor associated with low quality of life among impoverished people (Baumstarck, Boyer, & Auquier, 2015). Housing offers the foundational platform from which youth launch their trajectories towards non-street cultures. For the vast majority, having a place to call their own—a roof, a bed, a kitchen, a fridge and stove, a private washroom—was seen as a deep privilege, and as a significant foundation from which to regain a sense of citizenship and humanness.

Not surprisingly, the types of housing that young people held greatly influenced how their transition unfolded. Supported housing with roommates was helpful, because the price is affordable and formal supports are available, but organizational rules and conflicts with housemates often pushed youth to make premature exits into more costly and less secure market rent options. Supportive housing can also lead youth into a holding pattern where they find it challenging to move beyond basic stability by working towards personal goals and achieving mainstream markers of success. We found that the most effective supportive housing coupled support and guidance with opportunities for individual problem solving and room to learn from mistakes. Similarly, Gassman and Gleason (2011) found that youth-serving organizations need to be intentional about developing and promoting healthy mentoring relationships to create positive environments for staff and the youth being served. Living alone in market rent housing was rare for youth in our study because it is expensive, leaving most youth in market rent accommodations no choice but to find roommates. This strategy was most common among youth who were disconnected from service agencies. Further, it was the least stable because of conflicts with landlords (who were often exploitive) and roommates (who were wrestling with their own struggles).

> It was good; however, it turns out that the roommates I had, there was bad credit, all this stuff, and it just wasn't working out. They were ready, one of them in particular … just started being late for the rent and rent is dirt cheap. Come to figure out that that person is just a pathological liar altogether … Eventually, he was just not there. Eventually, the other roommate was not there, but because of the whole thing the landlord was giving us time to, you know, vacate the premises.

Establishing basic stability was essential for moving towards mainstream goals, and the loss of housing often derailed any forward momentum that youth had established. While having a place to stay provided a roof over one's head, it was only when youth began to feel that they had a sense of safety, peacefulness, hopefulness, and purpose that housing began to provide important psychological benefits. To varying degrees and amounts of time, this was true for the majority of participants—having their own place translated into feeling healthier, both physically and psychologically, happier, and more human.

For many, their present living arrangements felt like home. While providing a sense of freedom and independence (especially for those who have lived in shelters and supportive housing structures), apartments also allowed youth to feel more like a "person" than a "street kid." Having a stable space also empowered young people to reflect more on their future and reassured them that they were on the right track. One participant saw her apartment as "an anchor." Another stated, "It's weird, like, it really just goes from feeling like a box that you can hide in to a place that you can explore outwards from."

Numerous young people highlighted the importance of the mundane—having furniture, food in the fridge, the ability to take a shower or make a cup of coffee, access to technology such as video games, an Internet connection, and a phone—in allowing them to feel "normal" and "connected." For a few individuals, their apartments were safe spaces where they could privately and informally detox. The importance of routine also surfaced repeatedly in participants' accounts, particularly for those who seemed the most settled in their new lives. Again, these findings illustrate the critical role of emotional intelligence: how, over time, the youth consciously shifted from engaging in sporadic, and often risky, behaviour to developing self-control skills that gradually acknowledged the types of decisions needed to build stability in their lives.

> I like the routine. I learnt, it grew onto me; it's like I don't know what I would be doing now if I didn't have a routine. Probably be all over. I'd be lost, I'd be all over the place, but the routine it makes me more focused on what I'm looking at, right? What I'm watching for, what I'm trying to get at.

It appears that notions of routine not only tie into feelings of stability and security, but also establish forward momentum and a secure foundation from which to take on new responsibilities. As noted by Urwyler and colleagues (2015), routine plays a critical role in cognitive health status and in providing structure and momentum in everyday life.

While housing certainly had some positive elements for these youth, for many it was incomplete, and for the majority these benefits began to fade in the face of new forms of adversity. For many, the first apartment brought out feelings of insecurity regarding the skills for knowing how to live independently: how to shop, budget, cook, have friends, and deal with neighbours. There was a genuine fear of taking on too much at such a young age. One young man in a supportive housing program described wanting to take the next step but not "having a clue what people pay for like their normal house shit."

   In addition, it is important to note that having a place to stay was not sufficient for all participants to experience a sense of security and contentment. Indeed, for several in our sample, their current living space was not "home," but rather "a roof over [their] head." They felt the strain and anxiety of being independent: of having to find work, deal with bills and budgeting, handle housing and landlord issues, and manage their social life. As others have noted (Elliott & Canadian Paediatric Society, Adolescent Health Committee, 2013), this lack of comfort and security was particularly common among individuals who continued to deal with significant mental health and/or addiction issues. While independent living did provide an escape from the external world, and a place to heal and recover, some individuals were not yet at a stage where they could take advantage of such stability. Instead, these individuals tended to feel very disconnected from their environments and somewhat angry and frustrated with their position in life. In relation to issues of loneliness, depression, and post-traumatic stress disorder (PTSD), participants explained:

> I just noticed it's getting more; I'm more aware of it now as opposed to before. I was just really angry and pissed off. So, it wasn't like, you know what I mean. I didn't sit beside myself as much before 'cause I was always in the heat of this chaos and you know, whatever is going on.
>
>   I find, yeah, see for me I find it's more like my mental health is what really defines what goes on in the physical. You know what I mean? Like if I'm happy then most likely everything kinda falls together on its own. If I feel safe and independent and secure, I'm more likely to go pursue better things and jobs and do more positive, constructive things. You know what I mean? As opposed to if I'm fucking pissed off or sad or you know what I mean, just down and out and ... I find that that is where ... 'Cause you know I can have a place on my own, but if I'm constantly stressed out and pissed off or whatever, most likely things are gonna fall apart, right?

Most youth were caught at various points along this continuum—between the *positive* and *limited/limiting* aspects of housing. Points along this continuum are presented in the case vignettes in the next chapter.

"Mainstream" Acceptance

The third stage is broad and can last indefinitely as it is the stage in which youth work towards establishing a non-street life. Participants described this stage in terms of a "middle ground" where they were at times caught between their previous street lives and their current non-street environments. Many struggled to redevelop their sense of self to fit in with their new existence. This crucial period of trying to pull things together and move forward is probably the most challenging part of the transition out of homelessness. A good level of basic stability and having a goal or purpose (reason to try) in mind are crucial for any kind of success or building motivation for change in this stage.

> I think the biggest thing is I knew where I wanted to be and I knew the things I was supposed to do. But … I didn't like myself or really care about doing it until I got into a relationship and realized that it's not just me that I have to, to take care of. And at the time, taking care of me was something I didn't wanna do. So now I have to not only take care of myself for myself, but because of this other person and I have to take care of, not have to care or anything, but I want to take care of this other person and … and I wanna be happy and I want, you know, we have animals too; we have to take care of them and it, it's more of like a responsibility. I didn't have any responsibilities back then and, and so there's no point in, in taking care of myself. So, so I think the biggest thing has been just being, getting more responsibilities and having a reason to feel responsible about myself or someone else.

As others have found (Fortin, Jackson, Maher, & Moravac, 2015), a similar reflection process was experienced by a number of mothers in our study during which they realized that they had a responsibility to pull themselves together and become productive role models for their children (see Chapter 3). With focused determination, they gradually developed a positive view of themselves and their ability to be mothers, along with goals for the future.

> Well, I was in detox for like a month and a half and then I went to the CAMH thing [counselling project] and … I had to tell them my story or whatever

and I ended up flipping out; I was so angry, it all just burst. But ever since then, I don't know, it was just such a weight off my shoulders and then I could realize … that if I passed a mirror I would call myself ugly and stupid and stuff like that, and I realized I had been doing it forever and I made myself stop all that crap and my self-esteem is really good, especially getting into this new place.

As this young mother identified, self-esteem, a positive self-concept, and self-control (determination) played an important role in the transition process and were key elements of this particular transitional stage. Participants who had some success connecting to a socially valued role, like motherhood, often noted the pleasure and satisfaction of a redefined self-concept and identity, key elements of maturity. Furthermore, this shift in self-concept was reinforcing and created positive momentum for a number of participants as it gave them a sense of where they might fit into mainstream society.

Education and employment were also significant elements of one's identity that provided avenues towards mainstream acculturation. Most respondents were in school or had plans to attend. But the youth we interviewed have complicated lives that made focusing on education while dealing with other stressors (poverty, family stress, friend or partner drama, and mental and/or physical health issues) extremely challenging. In addition, a number of youth also had to manage numerous other barriers, such as learning disabilities and a dislike for school stemming from a history of conflicted experiences within the educational system.

Employment is also a critical component affecting the transition towards stability. Indeed, Nelson, Gray, Maurice, and Shaffer (2012) found that improvements in work and related life skills were associated with increased self-esteem and self-efficacy, and that these improvements predicted stable housing situations. Similarly, our study participants with a steady work history, reflecting strong self-control, tended to be particularly self-motivated and self-disciplined. However, the most common type of work for most youth in the study was low-wage service jobs. Participants tended to find this work boring and difficult to maintain given their complicated lives. As two participants note:

[On working at a "doggy daycare"] Yes, the work is good. Especially, I was doing full time but I cut back my hours to not so much 'cause it's like working in daycare; it's like Zen training, I swear to you, 'cause it's in the whole infrastructure that's where … you will get all the shit. If anything's going wrong, all the negative energy people will just like pile it.

And so because I had to make really tough decisions, like, well, do I work full time so I can retain my livelihood or do I try to keep going to school and just hope it figures out or something. Stay on OW [Ontario Works]. So there was a lot of tough decisions around that. And I still hope to keep doing my school and … take courses.

Managing friendship networks was also complicated during this transition stage. One of the most common struggles in our participants' lives involved their numerous attempts to distance themselves from street life and street communities. Taking self-control in their lives by removing themselves from street activities, such as drug misuse and petty thievery, was important for developing and maintaining a non-street status and signalled further developmental maturity. In addition, participants explained that, as they engaged more self-control by making changes in their lives, it became increasingly difficult to relate to friends who had not: "No, I don't think they [street friends] treat me any different and that's maybe, probably the issue, I don't know. I don't know what it is, it's just, they want to do the same things that we did back then and I don't want to do those anymore." Forging new friendships outside of the street context was an important marker of stability and positive influences in their new lives.

Lastly, romantic relationships were a complex terrain for the young people in our study. Having experienced neglect, abandonment, and abuse, the young people we spoke with often struggled with trust within their romantic unions. In addition, these relationships were further complicated by the fact that the romantic partners were often individuals who also had experienced trauma or were themselves transitioning away from homelessness:

I had met somebody in … the shelter system, at that time when I went to Vancouver as well. [It became a] relationship, and then we got together and …

at first we were separate, kind of doing our own separate things and finding our own places and everything like that. And then eventually both our situations fell apart. And then we came together and got a place together and, yeah, became a full-fledged relationship … And that was a problem and a half.

Trust was a prominent and reoccurring theme in the interviews, with a number of the young people discussing their "trust issues" and the ongoing difficulty they had believing in the people around them. In many instances, these trust issues could be linked back to the insidious, diffuse, and often hidden impact of trauma on a young person's perceptions and attachment to others (Cook et al., 2005). Problems with trust appeared to manifest at this stage in the exiting homelessness process because with more stability in their lives, young people were beginning to turn their attention to the task of establishing new, more long-term interpersonal connections across a number of domains (e.g., school, work, romantic). One direct way that problems with trust undercut stability and momentum during this stage was by destabilizing living arrangements with romantic partners. Fights and breakups were a common reason for the young people losing their housing.

Achievement

The fourth and final stage is the realization of lasting economic and social inclusion. It is a stage characterized by robust stability, the fulfillment of primary life goals, and the achievement of mainstream markers of success. No youth from our study could be classified as having reached this stage during the study period, and it is a level of stability and security that an unfortunate number of marginalized individuals never achieve, despite their best efforts. Mainstream society sends clear messages about who is acceptable. Indeed, "'marginalization' is not simply one thing, not just one status [e.g., homeless]. While an absence of economic resources may, to be sure, characterize a marginalized group, lack of knowledge, political rights and capacity, recognition and power are also factors of marginalization" (Jensen, 2000, p. 1). The following passage illustrates the sorts of structural barriers and contradictions that young people like our participants must overcome in order to reach this stage. It also illustrates the level of determination that some youth had developed in order to succeed:

No, that's actually one of the biggest problems, that's actually one of my biggest problems right now. Everyone else has money and I'm kind of sitting here broke and I don't want to hop on to the welfare boat. No, I just won't hop on to the welfare boat, you know? So, I don't know … Couldn't tell you where they get it sometimes. Some of them just have some money and some of them just don't. But right now, me not having money is my issue and it's really bothering me so … [And what makes you think you wouldn't want to go on welfare?] I wouldn't want to get comfortable on welfare. That's the thing. You know what I mean? My mom's been comfortable on welfare since I was born; you know, the apple doesn't fall far from the tree. And I tend to just … I'm really bad at saving money and I spend money on stupid shit. And I spend it fast, too. And if I had a job, don't they deduct the money I make from my welfare cheque anyways? So what would welfare really do for me? … You know, I'd have a cheque at the beginning of the month and then it'd be done. I'd probably spend that fast. And at least if I'm working for money I'd feel bad about spending the money; it's not just free income kind of thing, you know. I'm better off when I have paycheques kind of thing, so, I don't know, maybe.

FACTORS SHAPING THE TRANSITION THROUGH HOMELESSNESS

Within the four stages described above, there exists a range of forces that shape how individuals moved through the trajectories of their transition.

Consistent Support

One of the most striking findings from our data is the importance that participants attributed to informal personal supports—at first, particular service providers with whom they made connections, and later, usually one particular family member, but also boyfriends and girlfriends who acted as their best friend and primary support mechanism. In exploring the trajectories of our sample group members, episodes of happiness, health, and stability corresponded with participants feeling that they had one special individual in their lives whom they could count on. Dang and Miller (2013) also found that social supports provided by mentors enhance youth's adaptive functioning and may promote resilience. They argued that the use of natural mentors may be an important untapped asset in designing interventions to improve outcomes for homeless youth.

Conversely, at times when participants expressed strain and stress in their lives, they often lacked such a person. Clearly, one of the core dimensions of stability for these youth was the sense that there was someone in their lives to feel connected with and who both *cared about* and *cared for* them. This sense of belonging cannot be underestimated—it has a great impact on our participants' sense of self, health, and stability. For example, one study participant fell back into addiction and compromised his living situation when his brother, who was his key support, left the city to move to another part of the country.

A key finding is that the research participants who felt safe and supported had an individual in their lives who was consistent, who was present, and who provided unconditional love. As discovered in a previous study of street exiting (Karabanow, 2008), having someone in their lives who remained present during the inevitable ups and downs of growing up was a significant factor for youth feeling stable and healthy. The majority of the participants who made significant gains in their trajectory away from homelessness had such an individual, and we were surprised to note that those individuals tended to be family members. Regardless of the tensions and conflicts of the past familial relationship, participants repaired fractures in order to allow their family members back into their lives. This was most visible with our young mother participants and their relationships with their respective mothers. This rebonding provided participants with an important layer of support and stability. However, it is worth noting that many of these repaired family relationships continued to be complicated and to require significant effort and compromise to maintain. This dynamic is captured in the comic towards the end when the main character reconnects with his family but still feels conflict with his stepfather.

Stergiopoulos and colleagues (2014) also report the difficulties that individuals experienced during their transition of securing housing and living alone and note the critical role played by supports (both social and service supports) in assisting individuals during the early stages and when addressing difficulties, including lack of life skills and social isolation. Social supports provide an important buffer against stressful life events and were found to play a crucial role in promoting improvements in physical and psychological community integration, as well as quality of life. Further, as others have found (Dang & Miller, 2013; Gassman & Gleason, 2011) among those with previous experience in shelters or supported housing arrangements, those who had a strong working alliance with staff (service supports) were more likely to have improved outcomes in community integration (both physical and psychological) and in quality-of-life domains when they moved into stable housing.

Feelings of Belonging

When asked about their sense of community, the vast majority of study participants understood this concept solely in terms of the geographical space around their current independent living arrangement, and did not express any deep commitment to the setting or the people. For the most part, participants were living in high-rise apartments and seemed to connect with other residents only when there were visible similarities (such as another single parent or family with children). As such, participants generally did not express a sense of belonging within mainstream culture. The only evidence of experiencing membership in a local community came from those living in supportive housing structures with like-minded residents (i.e., single mothers). Although they typically linked the notion of community with their geographical surroundings, a number of youth felt a sense of community in other areas of their life—usually based on an activity they participated in or a group of people who had similar interests. There seems to be a connection between the youth who appear to be the most stable and those who have found a community with whom they identify.

Life and Social Skills

Other factors shaping the transition away from homelessness were basic life skills such as cooking, cleaning, and managing finances. Transitional housing programs were helpful in building these skills if youth did not already have them. Social skills could both facilitate and impede a transition into the mainstream, and therefore were also a significant factor. They were helpful in building support networks—outgoing and charismatic youth were good at getting the help of friends and social services. But they could also impede transitions to mainstream goals because the most social youth tended to stay connected with street-involved friends and acquaintances, thereby involving participants in interpersonal drama and conflict, and increasing the likelihood of returning to destructive activities like crime or drug misuse.

Being Ready

Notwithstanding external supports, many participants spoke of an internal and deeply personal decision-making process that signalled "being ready" to get off the street and live independently (this was also found in Karabanow et al.'s 2010 street-exiting study). Others spoke about "being willing to change" and take life more seriously at the current stage in their lives. So while conventional arguments within the homelessness literature call for increased government funding towards continued emergency shelter resources, which is no doubt important, there is also a need to acknowledge the role of self-control and individual agency in making choices that will support street exiting and healthy living post-street life. Personal identity and the extent to which youth ever identified with homeless life are important components of this internal orientation. Having aspects of a mainstream identity was framed as useful for pursuing mainstream goals. Of course this needed to be matched, once again, by self-control and determination, along with a sense of efficacy—a sense that they could in fact martial the internal and external resources to successfully pursue such goals.

Goal Setting and Routine

Goal setting was similarly significant. Goals were often helpful during the initial transition as they helped motivate young people. Overly ambitious goals, however, could be a liability because they can be a source of frustration. Similarly, expectations played a critical role in the transition. It was easier for youth to realize mainstream goals if they were able to develop *realistic* expectations about the future and come to terms with the monotonous, yet stabilizing and grounding effects of routine that often comes with mainstream daily life once the high-risk lifestyle of street life is given up. Indeed, a number of participants in our study spoke about how routine, despite its often boring rituals, enabled them to gain stability and a number of positive outcomes. For mothers, in particular, family routine, built through conscious self-control and other emotional intelligence skills, helped to preserve family integrity and to provide hope for the family to continue into the future.

Self-Control

As noted earlier, we found that self-control was associated with more mainstream success in our youth. Those who were able to identify goals and establish a focused action plan accomplished more. For example, one study participant who joined our study having just completed a methadone program and moved into supportive housing was determined to advance her education. By the end of the study period she was living in a stable housing situation, had finished upgrading her high-school education, and was well on her way to earning a college diploma.

As another example, one of the mothers reconnected with her child's father during the study and both agreed to engage in abuse counselling in an effort to meet the province's child protection requirements to re-engage as a family. The mother insisted on staying in supportive housing with her child to the end of her time limit (two years), yet ensured that the family got together regularly and that both parents focused on enhancing their parenting skills. The mother had very clear expectations of herself—that she complete high school and "never be on welfare." She had similarly high expectations of her partner if they were to remain a couple—that "he complete high school and get a job." By the end of the year, her determination (self-control) and resilience enabled the family to move into independent housing, and her work was recognized by the supportive housing staff, who asked her to give a speech at a fundraising event.

Coping

Another significant factor in the success of the young people we interviewed to make gains in stability had to with young people finding effective ways to cope and manage stress in their lives (all elements of emotional intelligence). This theme intersects with the finding that supportive people play a critical role throughout the street-exiting process by assisting youth with stress management and self-care. Beyond the support of others, participants also described important coping strategies such as strategies for making their living space feel calm and rejuvenating, spiritual practices, journalling, and music and art. This theme is captured in the comic when the main character, after a long day of disappointing news, puts on his headphones and begins to sketch. As noted previously in this section, poverty disconnects these young people from many of the consumerist ways to find pleasure and relieve stress (e.g., going out for dinner or a movie, taking a sunny vacation, going to the spa), and so it was important that respondents find other creative ways to create peace and pleasure in their lives on a limited budget. While these stress-relieving strategies were key to survival on the street, they often took on new meaning when youth found housing and new stresses began to emerge.

Hope

Embedded within the participants' personal reflection was an engagement in a sense of hope for the future. Despite the uncertainty and fragility of their transitions, the process of acquiring and sustaining housing gave many of the young people in our sample access to a new sense of self. Participants spoke of "not giving up" and maintaining the perspective that "things will get better," and suggested that civil society perceive them as "strong" and "resilient," with deep convictions to have a better life. They dreamed of finishing high school, entering university or college, finding a meaningful job, buying a house, and starting a family—all very mainstream and middle-class ideals that stem from traumatic and disadvantaged pasts. As one participant told us, "I would like to have a place to rent where maybe there's a piece of grass I can play with my kid on and like a street where they can ride their bike down the street or things like that, you know what I mean. Just normal shit that people take for granted, but I mean that's basically what I'm striving for at this point."

While present at different times to varying degrees, we also observed the fragility of this hope. Hopeful narratives proved difficult to sustain amid a myriad of structural and personal barriers that for a quarter of the youth we spent time with went so far as to send them back to street homelessness. Indeed, this ambiguity surrounding hope is further highlighted by the overall decline in our quantitative measure of hope over the one-year period.

CONCEPTUAL FOUNDATIONS

We end this chapter with two conceptual frames that underpin our findings. *Charting a path to adulthood* and *states of fragility* are key aspects to the transitions from street life to housing stability. Much of housing first practices have ignored both dynamics—the vast majority of its policies and applications have not involved youth populations directly, and there has been surprisingly little discussion in terms of this population's vulnerability and fragility within their trajectories.

Ambiguous Status as Adults

Deeply anchored within all of these findings is evidence that, unlike their stably housed counterparts, youth transitioning off the streets are forced simultaneously to address the challenges of emerging adulthood and overcome current and/or past trauma, without adequate supports. Our participants described lives in which they have had to "grow up much too fast." They have undergone deep and consistent trauma in their short lives only to be pushed out to become adults much too early. As one participant noted, she struggled with "not being ready" and not "having the supports" needed. Episodes of violence, abuse, neglect, and exploitation have strained their sense of childhood, forcing them to abandon some worlds to survive in others. As noted above, such youth are vulnerable developmentally.

The majority of these young people have had to survive on the street, find formal and informal supports, seek out employment, and subsequently locate stable accommodations, on their own. The normal trajectory for middle-class young, or "emerging," adults in North America is for these tasks to be taken up within the context of starting post-secondary education around nineteen years of age, with the support of caring parents. Our participants spoke of a very different trajectory, as they were forced to establish their adult life without the loving and caring support of their families.

There is also a deep contradiction within the developmental pathway. While they have been forced to become fully-fledged adults in terms of survival, they continue to be perceived as adolescents by civil society. Participants spoke of feeling overwhelmed and disrespected by the myriad of rules and structures at shelters and supportive housing settings, which infantilized them and ignored their developmental reality. As one young person explained, "Before I needed the help. Now I don't need the help. I don't need to be under one, two, three, five other laws beside our own 'cause you got a worker, the guy in charge of where you're at, their boss, their boss, and their boss ..." Moreover, landlords and employers rarely took them seriously due to their age and inexperience:

> I'm tired of being the bottom of the class. Our assistance can pay for like a thousand; me and [Curt] combined can pay for almost over a thousand dollars. So, we should be able to get a nice place with that, but the thing is we already went to look at a place and they already turned us down because of our age. [Curt]'s twenty, [Sarah]'s twenty-one, and I'm twenty-two, and they just turned us down. They're like, "We're not going to let you guys in here 'cause you're young."

Ironically, being forced to become an adult too soon places these youth at risk. When they are ready to become stable, formal systems struggle to accept them because they are not yet recognized as full adults.

The Fragility of Stability

One of the formal criteria for inclusion in our study was that participants needed to have been off the street for six months and be in what they perceived to be "stable living" accommodations (i.e., supportive housing and/or independent market accommodations). As such, this is a group of people who have already committed themselves to the difficult task of achieving housing stability and transforming their street identity into a non-street sense of self:

> It was ... on/off, on/off, like you know, I'd be stable for a little bit and then I'd go back to the shelter. I'd be in school for a little bit, then I couldn't do it anymore. And then have to go back to working or ... you know? Just like got chaotic. Like crazy, crazy, crazy. I was coming into myself as well.

What seems extremely telling is that, even as success stories, these youth struggle on a daily basis to maintain the basic stability that the reconstruction of their identity depends upon. Herrera, Jones, and Thomas de Benitez (2009) note that "street youths lack the resources with which to 'buy into' consumerist forms of subjectivity," and so must fashion their subjectivity through their internal struggles to maintain hope and persevere with their plans, and by seeking out external supports (by way of youth services and family).

But for the majority of our sample, they *just barely* remain stably housed. One of the core themes of our work, then, is that the majority of these young people remain in a very fragile state during their transition into non-street-based emerging adults. Canadian public health researcher Karen Boydell thoughtfully articulates this complex entanglement of identity:

> Homelessness means a loss of social identity—loss of permanent address, work, school, relationships, and place to call one's own. On a personal level, homelessness can mean a loss of self. Homelessness involves much more than not having a place to live. Individuals often lose their sense of identity, self-worth, and self-efficacy. (Boydell, Goering, & Morrell-Bellai, 2000, p. 26)

Many of our respondents feared losing their market rent apartments or supportive housing units if they "messed up," becoming ineligible for social assistance or disability allowances if they entered the formal or informal job market, or not having the personal and professional supports in place that could "prop them up" in times of despair. One participant described his day-to-day life as feeling like he is "treading water," or moving "one step forward, two steps back." For many, there is a consistent fear that they will once again be homeless if certain situations arise (such as mental health flare-ups, loss of employment, loss of assistance, or renewed struggles with addictions). Moreover, there was a sense from numerous participants that their current lives could change at any moment, and that they had little control over maintaining their current stability. For example, one participant explained that during a bus strike in her town, she risked losing a subsidized daycare spot for her child and falling behind in school due to the long commute to both locations and regulations stipulating that she or her child could not be absent from either institution for more than a few days. Another young woman highlighted the unlucky combination of having a disability and being consistently stuck in casual, low-paying employment:

That's one of my biggest worries is that if I try, if I try to get a job or try to get off disability I'm just going to screw myself over … I have all my medical bills to pay and so it's just not something that easy that I can just get off of because … it's not like I can just live off dumpstering [finding thrown-away food in dumpsters] and live in a closet. I have [a] few hundred dollars a month in medical bills to pay for being diabetic. So I really want to be able to get a job in the future that does pay, that does have benefits, what's it called, have a health plan [health insurance that would cover medication and particular treatments not part of universal coverage in Canada].

It is this feeling of insecurity that underlies our participants' daily lives. As many of them suggest, their stability can change overnight. The result is the feeling that they have very little control over their life circumstances. The following three participants demonstrate the fear and anxiety that result as these feelings of disempowerment shape day-to-day existence:

I'm just scared that it's gonna, I don't know, something's gonna give out. I just, I always have this feeling something's gonna give out, like it's gonna happen again. I'm just gonna get homeless again or something bad's gonna happen. I'm put in a situation, something's gonna happen, you know?

Just because my diabetes is really, really fragile, and even the last year I've thought, I had really bad dips in blood sugar … I used to be able to not test my blood sugar for two years and be fine. But now it's like if I don't test it for a day then I could … get kind of shitty with it. So it's really fragile and I'm scared that if I slip and if I miss an appointment and I get weird and don't have my insulin or don't have my testing supplies … I'm just so always close to it, this lovely anxiety that I'm just … even when I lost my birth certificate I was like so now I can't cash my cheque. My disability cheque, and that was just kind of like this "Oh God, it's all gonna happen again." And I just have this major fear if I lose, like I said, losing my wallet, could end up … could actually kill me, and that's like a fear. Like as soon as I go back to it and just slowly don't take care of myself that I'm gonna get sick and die. And it's just like somebody with severe anxiety in this system—it's just constantly trying to catch up and not be drowned in it.

I'm always scared, each month at the end of the month, I'm always scared that assistance isn't gonna come through and pay rent. I'm always terrified of that because I've been cut off assistance without my knowledge twice in the last three years.

One of our core discoveries is that, despite the fact that members of our research population are perceived as successes, they experience their worlds as being highly stressful, overwhelming, fragile, and draining. Much like Forchuck, Ward-Griffin, Csiernik, and Turner (2006) found when exploring the experiences of psychiatric consumer-survivors related to housing, many of our youth lived in fear, worried about losing control of basic human rights, finding ways to hold on to and create relationships, identifying supports and seeking services, and obtaining personal space and place. While service providers and the general public perceive these young people as less at risk, new layers of risk emerge as a consequence of their shaky transitions towards stability. As one participant eloquently noted, in the context of this fragility, there were often deep tensions about what it meant to be stable, which led to her feeling uncertain about her "progress" and "what it all means."

CONCLUSION

It is not surprising that our participants, as a particular segment of the youth population who have transitioned out of basic homelessness, continue to describe their current lives in terms of fragility and instability. Clearly, while housing in itself does not shape these young people's sense of stability, it definitely influences feelings of health, happiness, and security. There are numerous interrelated factors at play that allow participants to regain a sense of citizenship, or feelings that they are part of mainstream society. The complex and nuanced pathways from street to mainstream are fraught with uncertainty and struggle. The journey occurs during the early twenties: a time fraught with numerous developmental struggles (regarding identity, instability, self-focus, and feeling in-between), but also an age filled with possibilities. The following chapter, through case scenarios, further elucidates these conceptual dimensions.

CHAPTER 3

Working Towards Stability

In this chapter we zoom in, taking a detailed look at four qualitative case studies that shed additional light on the stages of the exiting process and that help to illustrate its complexity. Three of these case studies illustrate common pathways that underlie the broad quantitative findings summarized at the beginning of the chapter. The fourth case study describes the experience of a young mother, a group with a distinct set of experiences and one captured largely in Halifax, where a relatively large proportion of youth in this situation were interviewed.

A DIFFICULT ROAD

The goal of the larger longitudinal study was to articulate pathways out of street spaces and sociocultural contexts using qualitative and quantitative measures. In addition to gathering demographic data, young people were asked a series of standardized questions during each interview that allowed us to track their well-being and the well-being of the sample as a whole over the course of the year. Along with participant demographics, the following measures were used: (1) the Self-Concept Clarity Scale to evaluate the role of identity cohesion; (2) the Community Integration Scale, which taps psychological (belongingness) and behavioural (activities) components of community participation/involvement; (3) the brief World Health Organization Quality of Life Scale (WHOQOL-BREF), (4) the Mental Health Continuum-Short Form (MHC-SF); and (5) Snyder's cognitive measure of hope (see Table 2). To address the exploratory question about

TABLE 2 Means (M), standard deviation (SD), and within-group effect sizes (Cohen's d) for clinical and functional outcomes for participants in exiting street life study ($n = 51$)

Outcome Variable	T1		T2		T3		T4		d1	d2	d3
	M	SD	M	SD	M	SD	M	SD			
CIS	3.94	1.58	3.75	1.63	3.58	1.64	3.45	1.64	-.14	-.24	-.31
SOB	13.90	3.20	13.19	4.35	12.83	3.39	12.71	3.76	-.13	-.24	-.25
FS	44.47	7.32	43.27	9.22	42.15	8.00	40.19	11.74	-.18	-.39*	-.58*
SC	35.04	10.85	34.33	11.33	34.97	9.43	35.42	9.79	-.08	-.01	.04
QOL	88.30	11.97	86.05	11.25	84.65	12.40	86.33	12.70	-.20	-.41*	-.19
MHQ	45.72	11.12	43.76	9.49	42.62	11.46	46.61	11.76	-.22	-.42*	.09

Note: d1 = effect size between time 1 and time 2; d2 = effect size between time 1 and time 3; d3 = effect size between time 1 and time 4; CIS = Community Integration Scale; SOB = Sense of Belonging Scale; FS = Future Scale; SC = Self-Concept; QOL = Quality of Life; MHQ = Mental Health Questionnaire.

*p < .05

the extent to which mental health, community participation, self-concept, and quality-of-life change over a one-year period, we conducted paired-samples t-tests and within-group effect sizes (Cohen's d) reported for changes between (1) baseline and four months, (2) baseline and eight months, and (3) baseline and twelve months (see Table 2).

In terms of demographic differences, we found that females had spent less time on the streets than males (mean 18.73 vs. 32.79 months), but they emerged as equivalent to males across the domains of well-being. No differences were noted as a function of sexual identity. Generally, youth in independent housing (as opposed to supported housing models) reported spending less time engaged in community activities, had a lower quality of life, and struggled to a greater extent with mental health challenges and distress. Interestingly, *quantitative* differences did not emerge as a function of study location; however, *qualitative* narratives regarding motherhood were more prominent in Halifax, while those regarding ethnic and racial diversity were more evident in Toronto. Over time, we did not find a pattern of improvement on quantitative indicators, as one might expect of young people who had found housing and who were moving away from the adversity of homelessness. Analysis of key mental health and well-being indicators suggested a modest decline over the one-year period, with several indicators registering some improvement in the second half of the year in mental health and quality of life. Overall, these quantitative results painted a picture of declining hope and valleys of reduced quality of life and mental well-being, which underscore the strain experienced by young people trying to exit from homelessness. These quantitative results also show that the transition off the streets, while different from life on the streets, presents significant challenges of its own that negatively affect an already stressed and vulnerable group.

CASE STUDIES: THREE TYPES OF PATHS AND MOTHERHOOD

What was broadly evident in the quantitative data becomes more complex and nuanced in the narratives of the youth we engaged. This work spoke to the manner in which such complex transitions are in many ways better captured and understood qualitatively. These narratives, as suggested in

Chapter 2, tended to reflect a long, cycling, and somewhat demoralizing process of transition. Many described an initial burst of hope and optimism upon leaving the streets, followed by a long and challenging path towards a meaningful and financially independent life. This period was also a time when young people felt the isolation of cutting off old social networks, and distress as many began to reflect on past trauma.

Across the fifty-one narratives, we found that most of the youth's experiences of transitioning away from homelessness could be described in terms of three key stages: *an initial turning point*; *basic stability but limited forward momentum*; and *looking to the future and beginning to achieve broader life goals*. Using these stages, we were then able to cluster our participants into three general groups based on the progress they made throughout their transition process of exiting homelessness during the year that we spent with them. What became very clear was that a one-year time frame did not allow for a meaningful articulation of a full process of transition (if and when that might occur). The first group (*struggling to get stable*) included participants who found themselves cycling in and out of the first stage of transition. These young people experienced a turning point and decided to leave the streets, but they could not establish basic stability during the year they spent with us. Youth in the second group (*stable but stuck*) had managed to achieve basic stability by returning to their families or finding affordable or transitional housing, but they struggled to get beyond basic stability. These young people were stable but reported feeling stuck and disillusioned. Our third group (*beginning to meet goals*) included participants who had entered the third stage. They were experiencing some successes in their personal and professional goals, such as going back to school, securing employment, pursuing artistic projects, volunteering, and improving relationships. This third stage often had its own momentum where successes in these domains invigorated youth and helped propel them forward.

In choosing the four case studies, we employed a consensus process to identify participants (pseudonyms are used here) whose interview material provided sufficient depth and breadth to represent common trajectories throughout the process of exiting from homelessness. As a result, four participants—three single individuals and one mother—were purposively chosen from the larger group of participants.

Dean—Struggling to Get Stable

Dean was eighteen years old when we first interviewed him, and his street involvement had begun years earlier when he started running away from group home and foster care placements. At the time of this first interview, Dean was living in an apartment with his girlfriend—an upgrade from some of the run-down and chaotic "party houses" where they had stayed as they finished off a summer of sleeping in a park with a group of friends. Unfortunately, this apartment stay did not last and Dean struggled to maintain basic stability over the year we were interviewing him. While in the apartment, Dean and his girlfriend supported themselves through social assistance and some criminal activity, but neither was confident about next steps. As demonstrated by the interview transcript below, Dean was ambivalent about low-wage employment and going back to school as viable pathways out of homelessness. He described a number of complex justifications for his skepticism, including limited success with those pathways in the past and bureaucratic barriers, along with low motivation, anger problems, and uncertainty about the payoff over the long term of mainstream pathways out of homelessness, particularly when compared to the more immediate rewards of criminal involvement:

I: In terms of this sort of moving towards getting a job and getting back into school sort of, how is that process going? And where do you see yourself in the process? Are you kinda getting sort of mentally sorted out and ready to go, or is it more practical stuff?

D: I'm very bad at putting a foot down and going forward with it. And there are still a couple of things that I need. I need my ID and … I can't get my ID until I go to the ID clinic.

I: How do you feel about the pathway you are on right now?

D: I really, really do wanna veer off, but it's like I know if I do, I don't know. I know if I stay on the track where I'm going, I know exactly what's in store for me. But if I veer off I don't know what's in store for me and I know it's positive, but at the same time I've never seen that positive outcome so … to me it … for all I know it doesn't exist. But I know it exists. I know it's there. But it's like … my brain just doesn't wanna pull through to me. Like OK, time to fucking grow up, go do your shit, you know, get on top of things ... [With the crime stuff] I know about and I know what's gonna happen is like right there. It's a hundred percent for sure and it's like in the next week. You know?

Later in the interview Dean added:

I'm [missing] too many credits. That's why I always weigh things. That's why criminal [behaviour] looks so much better and easier. 'Cause I have no credits. And I'm really lazy when it comes to school work, literally.

Dean's comments about being lazy fully acknowledge his lack of motivation as a barrier to exercising self-control in his life. At the same time, they also reflect a tendency for homeless young people to blame themselves for their situation and minimize the role played by other structural and institutional factors in abandoning vulnerable youth during a time of need. Dean's struggle with stability, including his problems with motivation and anger, could be understood as part of a complex interplay of factors that include trauma and anger from neglectful and abusive early home environments and negative contact with child protection services. Drug abuse and addiction, while initially engaged as coping strategies but eventually resulting in further trauma, also play a prominent role, along with the lack of support and mentoring from both social and service stakeholders. In talking about his lack of motivation, Dean comments:

D: And smoking [weed] doesn't help at all. Makes me more lazy ... I used to take like Ritalin and Adderall and Dexedrine and all that shit, and then I eventually stopped taking it, and as soon as I stopped taking it I started smoking weed. I'm very angry ... an easily irritable person. And when I smoke weed, I will tell jokes, like it's all jokes ... I was way angrier when I was a kid. Like I was psychotic when I was a kid. Like seriously. That's why they kept me on pills.

I: Right. And was there stuff in your life that was sort of part of that?

D: Just like being abandoned by a family. They're supposed to be, you know, loving and caring, like forever, da-de-de-dah, for some fucking CAS [Children's Aid Society] and business, pretty much, I'm being run by them.

My whole life I've just … wanted to be free … It sounds really cliché but I've just wanted to not be bossed around. Because … when I got my first charge in group homes they pretty much made it so that I couldn't, I couldn't do anything. I have to do exactly what they say or I go to jail. I AWOL'd a long time ago. And just stayed away. And it just worked. It just worked. And ever since then I just been, I been more clear-headed.

Dean's comments illustrate the complex ways that various factors interconnect and play out over time to shape the direction of a young person's life. They also underscore the key role played by *self-perception of competencies* and *self-regulation* in youth development in terms of individual decision making about engagement in learning and in goal-oriented daily life activities (Bronson, 2000; Nader-Grosbois, 2007).

Shortly after our first interview, Dean and his girlfriend lost their apartment and had to move into the one-bedroom apartment of some friends. This arrangement quickly soured and Dean and his girlfriend had to move again. After the move, Dean and his girlfriend broke up, in part because he was continuing to use crystal meth. Dean wanted to quit but was struggling: "I'm more [held off] from it, but when I do get into certain areas and certain, around certain people … then it triggers it. And it doesn't stop on the triggers. It's not like I can be like, oh yeah, hey, buddy. And then just be like, oh yeah, I'm gonna go home."

After the breakup, Dean went to jail for theft but managed to hold on to his apartment. Unfortunately, when he got released he returned to find that his roommate had moved out and he was not able to pay for the apartment on his own. After losing his place, Dean stayed in hotels and couch surfed. At the time of our last interview, Dean was bouncing between a hotel and a friend's father's house.

Importantly, during the year we were interviewing Dean, he had almost no connections with youth-sector social service agencies, and no family member or supportive adults in his life. In the larger sample, a key factor separating those who were able to maintain stability from those who were not appeared to be the presence or absence of emotional and practical/mentoring support from a stable individual like a parent or caseworker. Tozer and colleagues (2015) had similar findings. Indeed, youth partici-pants stressed that having personal goals and ties to social networks, along with supportive family and role models, and safe and stable housing were key factors in being resilient in giving up drugs. Sadly, support appeared to be worsening for Dean as his current trajectory was threatening his relationships with his more stable friends:

> **D:** We [old friends] don't really get along doing the same things.
>
> **I:** What are those things that you like to do that they're maybe not into or vice versa?
>
> **D:** To be quite honest, I like to do crime because it's easy money. But I realize I, I don't like doing time, I don't like sitting in jail. So I've been working on slowly, you know, fixing, getting, getting a job kinda thing. But [my roommate and her friend] kinda like called me up and that. It's like, "We're making like a lot of money in like three seconds." It was just crook money.

Dean describes how he is losing touch with his more stable friends as he becomes more involved in crime, but his comments also illustrate his ambivalence about his increasing criminal involvement—he knows that he is risking jail time, which he detests, but given his deep material need and lack of support, the lure of quick money is just too strong.

Overall, Dean's experiences highlight some key themes shared among those youth in the sample who struggled to establish basic stability. They also reflect Dean's self-reported mental well-being scores (quality of life, mental health, and hope), all of which remained fairly low with little change throughout the year (see Figure 1). In particular, his narrative illustrates the insidious, widespread, and long-term impact of childhood trauma from both family and public services (whose mission it is to protect) on multiple dimensions of life. In addition, his narrative reflects the destabilizing impact of drug abuse, the undercutting influence of hopelessness and resignation, and the consequences of limited emotional support and mentoring from stable adults.

Marcus—Stable but Stuck

Marcus' narrative captures themes that were common among individuals who had achieved basic stability over the course of the year, but who struggled to progress further. At his first interview Marcus had recently

FIGURE 1 Trajectory of select mental health and well-being indicators for case study participants

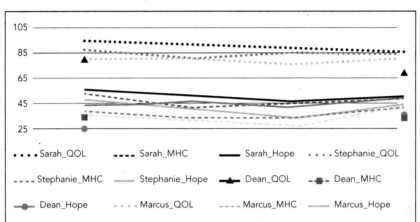

Note: QOL = Quality of Life; MHC = Mental Health Continuum.

moved into a market rent apartment, but he was eventually forced out of the apartment by a harassing and overly strict landlord:

> Yeah, I was smoking cigarettes on the front porch and one day he came by and he screamed at me for doing it, and I'm like, "I'm outside. I throw my cigarette butts in the garbage—what's your problem?" And I just told him, stop talking to me basically ... He was saying stuff like I smoked weed and how that was horrible and stuff. And he was calling me a drug dealer ... 'cause I had ... well, he had had big issues with people coming over to my house and there's nothing wrong to having someone over at your place ... I think for a couple of nights I had someone stay over and, and he said I wasn't paying for another person, how they can't stay at all and ... he's gonna charge them with trespassing. It was really ridiculous. He was just picking on me because I was young. The other tenants were in their forties or fifties.

The experience of dealing with a difficult landlord was common among participants, regardless of their stage in the trajectory, and was a significant threat to stability. Marcus' mental health was precarious during this time and he described suffering from psychosis, serious depression, and suicidal thoughts: "Yes it's, it's very depressing. I've never been this depressed in my life, actually. Yes. It's a little bit better, but for a while there I was contemplating suicide every day." This period of distress was one in a long history of ups and downs, including an incident where Marcus was arrested during an episode of psychosis, which was adjudicated through a mental health court (leaving him with a criminal record).

After leaving his apartment, Marcus cycled back into the emergency youth shelter system before moving into their transitional housing program. This move ushered in a period of stability and improved mental health and well-being. Through an emergency youth shelter Marcus was connected with a number of caseworkers, including one working with a specialized mental health program for street-involved young people. This was also a time when Marcus' parents were struggling with their own financial and mental health problems, and so were unable to provide much assistance to their son. The social service workers played a central role in assisting Marcus to gain overall stability and stabilized mental health. Indeed, practical supports (concrete services/assistance, mentoring, etc.) and emotional supports were key factors in promoting stability among our sample group. In addition, affordable and transitional housing programs played a critical role in promoting stability among participants—not only because of their affordability compared to market rent, but also because of their established links with services. Ojeda and colleagues (2016) also note the critical need for services that are age-specific for transition-age youths and that engage youths in the planning and delivery of services.

Along with these supports, Marcus was motivated to exit homelessness and had fairly realistic goals—namely a steady paycheque and a place he could call his own: "I don't wanna end up in [the adult shelter system], you know, I'm getting older. And I gotta get my, my shit in order. Do my trades, make eighty bucks an hour eventually. And ... maybe buy a house." However, despite his motivation, like other youth in the sample, Marcus faced a number of significant barriers to achieving his goals. While some barriers were related to Marcus' specific circumstances (criminal records, limited work experience, depression and anxiety), others related to the times and community context (e.g., narrow youth employment opportunities related to high unemployment rates, long waits for permanent subsidized housing, and inadequate supports for dealing with intellectual and mental health disabilities).

While Marcus did have a short-term employment contract working in an emergency shelter, his limited options and complex needs also meant that he spent a considerable amount of time at home "watching TV, smoking pot, and feeling down." Feelings of depression and hopelessness were a major risk factor that threatened the well-being and motivation, not only of Marcus but even those with less-complex needs in our study at this stage (*stable but stuck*). These feelings also were reflected in Marcus' self-reported mental well-being scores (quality of life, mental health, and hope), which, while higher than Dean's and improving somewhat during visit three, returned to the starting point by year-end (see Figure 1). These negative feelings often created a debilitating cycle of failure and hopelessness, a situation made worse by long waitlists for youth mental health services, particularly for one-on-one help. Dawson and Jackson (2013) also identify a number of significant barriers to service use among homeless youth, including lack of knowledge, provider attitudes, financial constraints, and inappropriate environments. Yet, while Marcus was fairly passive during his experience and while in the transitional housing program, he used art as a means of self-expression and coping. Indeed, art was a valuable coping tool, providing affirmation through visible achievement for many youth in our study, whose creative outlets included visual art, poetry, music, and dance. While evidence is relatively new in this area, it is growing and does support the role of art in mental health. For example, Brady, Moss, and Kelly (2017) have found that one form of art, art therapy integrated into mental health services, brings about improved quality of life and individual support. They also note its critical role as a non-verbal intervention.

Stephanie—Beginning to Meet Goals

Stephanie's story reflects the third stage, one of positive forward momentum. Throughout the course of the study, Stephanie showed incredible determination and managed to get herself to a point where she was moving towards her personal goals and beginning to feel a sense of positive momentum in her life. When we met Stephanie, she was in a methadone program and had just moved into supportive housing for young people exiting homelessness. By the end of the study period she was living in a stable housing situation, had finished upgrading her high-school education, and was well on her way to earning a college diploma. Stephanie described her typical day as one involving a good deal of routine that provided structure, set priorities, and built momentum, making it easier to persist:

> I get up probably six thirty every day and I go to school, usually to three ... I have class four days a week; Fridays I don't have class ... So when I have class I usually go to school and then go home, and once a week I have to meet with my worker, so sometimes I have to go home and my worker will be there. I go to the gym sometimes, too, and basically I do homework and go to bed, and start the whole thing over again, and I'm not liking it right now [laughs]. But it's good because I don't need time to breathe right now—if I have time to breathe, I'll be smoking. It's good because I think I know the methadone helps a lot with cravings and stuff for drugs, but I know when I have too much idle time is when I either slip into some sort of depression and sleep my day away or I start slipping.

Her stable routine of busyness, engaging self-regulation and success, helped her to see herself in a new way, and provided her with a new sense of accomplishment and self-worth:

> My high point, I guess going to school, that's huge, that's fucking huge. I never thought I'd do that, 'cause now I'm going to be a professional, I can't be fucking around, you know. Especially going to school for what I'm going to school, if I actually get into this field and stuff I'd be the talk of the town, the social worker on crack, you know [laughs]. So I think ... it's almost like I've put myself in this position so that I couldn't screw up kinda thing, but it's also good because I do stress out some days, and ... I have a network of people now that I never knew, and I have stuff to do that I never—like what would I do if I wasn't in school? And I don't really see it as big, but a lot of people are like, "Wow, you're doing good considering what I know you as," and I don't see it as much as other people see it, but I'd say that's something I've achieved, starting school, 'cause I still have to finish it.

A major theme in Stephanie's narrative was the importance of finding supportive people and the right kind of supported living arrangement. The main supports in her life were her psychiatrist and a caseworker who had been with her from the beginning of her time on the street. It is notable that Stephanie was one of the few youth with routine access to one-on-one counselling with a psychiatrist. Her caseworker had helped her into drug treatment and supportive housing, and was a consistent source of guidance and support throughout the year we were speaking with Stephanie:

> So I went to treatment, just to prove [to] people that I was doing better, but I had no intention of getting sober at the time, and then I went to another sober house through [an agency]—the lady that's my social worker has known me since I walked into [that house] until now right, so—and she's always like, "If you wanna get sober, I have a place for you to go" pretty much … Okay, so then I got kicked out of that house for using again, and I was living with my sugar daddy and I got really fucked up. And I ended up talking to a doctor and getting on methadone, and my doctor's actually friends with my social worker, so she contacted my social worker, told her I was sober and stuff, and then my social worker got me a place—so the place I live in now is still through [that same agency], but it's harm reduction, so if you happen to fuck up, you're not gonna get kicked out of it, right? Which is funny 'cause I haven't screwed up since I've been there, but if you put me in a sober house I get high [laughs] … Yeah. And it was good, because … I felt like, I'm gonna have something this stable? Because living in those other houses I felt like I was walking on eggshells … I can't even be honest with people because if I need help I can't reach out for it because I'm not supposed to be doing what I'm doing, so I need the help for what I'm doing, you know what I mean?

Stephanie's comments highlight the particular value of having someone to provide unconditional love and support through the inevitable ups and downs and cycles of transitioning away from homelessness. As others have noted (Hudson, Nyamathi, & Sweat, 2008), youth's ability to rehabilitate their lives depends on trusting and engaging relationships, often with adult service providers. Indeed, such support enabled Stephanie's *self-control*, *determination*, and *autonomy*, not the agency's rules, to make the decision to curb her drug use. At the same time, despite her successes, Stephanie's long history of trauma and victimization had a lasting impact on her well-being. One way this trauma manifested itself was in its powerful and lasting impact on her sense of trust, which made it difficult for her to maintain personal relationships:

> I've never had a stable group of friends growing up or anything, because I moved around so much. Everybody that I liked, helped, or cared about or anything has fucked me over … yeah, fucked me over, smashed my face against the wall. Like everybody. Even today I have the worst time trusting people; especially I have a really hard time in relationships and stuff, like intimate relationships, and even keeping a relationship. Sometimes I'll ignore my friend for like four days. I don't even know why I do it, but I have little habits … just in case you don't care, I don't care kind of thing.

The insidious impacts of trauma and victimization were commonly reported by the research participants. The young people we spoke with described how their problems with trust often led to unstable and stress-ful personal relationships that could be both socially and emotionally destabilizing. Stephanie credits her successful transition to *her choice* to distance herself from street- and drug-involved friends, demon-strating another relationship management theme common within the sample group:

> Basically I cut off, I don't talk to anybody. The day I walked out of that house with that backpack on, I never went back. I never talk to anybody, I never phone anybody, nothing. It's gone, and I think that's the best decision I made in my life. The hardest part is getting rid of people that you've known for so long—even though you guys are kinda fucked-up friends, they're still people that you care about and you see every day. [That process] was so hard. It's feeling like you're outside yourself and everything you know is wrong, but you don't even know where you're going. It's this fucking lost feeling, but a part of me knew if I just did it, that better things would happen kind of thing. And that's why when I relapsed, I started injecting opiates and stuff, I was so disappointed in myself and I was so like fuck this, because if I went through

all that shit and lost all these people and just left everything—I left, I had a cat, I left my apartment—I left everything and to go into this life and then I end up fucking it up, so I felt like I was a piece of shit, right? And then, I guess I proved that, and then I had no other choice but to get sober, 'cause I was so sick.

Stephanie's comments do an excellent job of capturing the dilemma faced by young people when it comes to managing their friendships. The peers who young people meet on the street can be an important source of support and understanding given their shared experience, but they can also be a pathway back to risky and destabilizing behaviours like drug use and criminal involvement.

In addition to continued problems with trust in old and new personal relationships, Stephanie experienced feelings of anxiety and depression and struggled to maintain her recovery in the face of school-related stress and the challenges of living in shared accommodations. Her experiences highlight that even the study participants who were doing well were often close to the edge, with only limited, newly formed safety nets to catch them if they slipped or experienced an unexpected structural shock such as a job loss or illness. The constant ups and downs of exiting from homelessness often led to feelings of ambivalence and disappointment: "So it's good. But it sucks 'cause I, I obviously feel hell of a lot better than I felt a year ago, but if you asked me a year ago how I would feel now, I think it would be so much better than what it is. Because you think it always is better than what it is but … I guess it is what it is, right? It's life, right?" In this comment Stephanie highlights how exiting homelessness can be a much more challenging and drawn-out process than youth anticipate. It is quite possible that this reality is the explanation for the declining hope captured by our quantitative analysis.

In addition to managing the stresses and emotional ups and downs, Stephanie also faced the lasting impact of a criminal record, mostly for drug and administrative charges. Criminal records are a serious barrier to employment. This is particularly true for the many young people in the sample who were interested in working in the social service sector, due to the common use of a comprehensive "vulnerable records checks" (which includes police contacts for mental-health-related issues and non-conviction records) used to screen those wishing to work with vulnerable populations like children and youth:

> So I finished school. I've been working on getting my pardon. Getting a pardon done 'cause I might have a problem with that next year with school. He [a person in the news] kept saying to his placement, "Oh, I'll get it, I'll get it." And that's what I did with my placement last year. Because of my records. So, I'm going through a pardon so if worse comes to worst, next year I won't do my placement; I'll have to wait till the year after.

Stephanie's experiences help to highlight some of the main themes we identified in the experiences of youth who managed not only to maintain basic stability over the year of the study, but to begin to experience success in their personal and professional goals. Her experiences also reflect her self-reported mental well-being scores (quality of life, mental health, and hope), which remained fairly stable throughout the year (see Figure 1). At the same time, her narrative demonstrates the critical role played by supportive housing and trusting caseworker support in successful transitions. It also highlights the ongoing challenges and struggles that even the most successful young people experience in managing the long-term consequences of homelessness, such as the lingering impacts of trauma and the limiting effects of a criminal record. Stephanie's story also points out the very human wish to, in turn, become a helper for others. Such responses can challenge the sense of helplessness that often accompanies trauma and assist Stephanie in building a sense of control in her life.

Sarah (Mom), Tyler (Son), and Randy (Partner/Father)

The discussion so far has focused on the experiences of three youth illustrating the common themes that characterize the trajectories through the exiting homelessness process. We now turn to a fourth case study to highlight the unique experiences and common themes of an important subgroup within the study, the young mothers—four from Toronto and nine from Halifax.

The mothers in our study had similar demographics to mothers in other youth homelessness research in that they shared family histories of violence, poverty, social isolation, and a lack of informal support, which contributed to their street experiences (Gültekin, Brush, Baiardi, Kirk, & VanMaldeghem, 2014; Karabanow & Hughes, 2013). Further, while many of the mothers in our study moved through similar stages to those encountered by the youth without dependants, they also faced a number of challenges unique to the role of parent. Pregnancy was a common tipping point that caused the mothers in our study to either take action to *exit* street life or to be kicked out of home and *enter* street life. A mother's attention was never entirely self-focused. Instead, it was constantly divided between her own needs and those of her child. Yet, as others have found (David, Gelberg, & Suchman, 2012), we observed that the physical, emotional, and financial difficulties faced during periods of homelessness greatly stressed mothers' capacity to parent. Despite this, recognizing that these mothers had little control over their environment, they were hesitant to seek—or accept—assistance for fear of drawing attention from child welfare. And while child protection services played an ongoing role with many mothers in our study, some mothers persevered, following all agency directives in order to keep their children. The experience of being a parent while homeless created a pivotal turning point for some mothers, who, in turn, made a conscious decision to become a responsible, loving parent. They took action not only to address their own needs (housing, substance use, health care, etc.) but those of their child as well. Such a turnaround demanded in-the-moment and continued commitment. One mother in our study, Sarah, showed particular resilience.

During our first interview with Sarah, we learned that she had been fifteen years old when her mother's marriage ended. She then moved in with her boyfriend's family, but after being kicked out, the couple was forced to start couch surfing with friends. Later that year, Sarah became pregnant and the delivery triggered a hospital visit by child protection services. Being afraid that she might lose her baby, she created a story to accommodate what she believed to be the law.

> **S:** Well, I was too young to get on social assistance, right, so and Randy [partner], he was old enough, he was nineteen when we had Tyler, so he was allowed to be on assistance because we couldn't find jobs and stuff, right?

So he was on assistance but I wasn't allowed to live with him because I was underage and he wasn't allowed to be my guardian where he's my spouse. So when I had Tyler I had to tell them [child protection] that, 'cause when you're under I think it's eighteen or something, they come and there's a social worker that comes when you have a baby and asks you how you are going to support them financially. And I had to tell them that Randy was going to take him and that I wasn't going to live with him.

I: Was that true?

S: No ... 'cause I wasn't allowed to live with Randy ... so I had to tell them that Randy was going to take him and I was just going to go somewhere and just visit him, but that wasn't true—I lived there. But when I told her [child protection] that, she told me that I shouldn't have to sign my rights over to Randy ... and she helped me advocate for social assistance so I could live with them. It took so long but we were able to live together.

However, while protocol eventually allowed the family to live together, family violence soon surfaced, resulting in child protection once again taking control.

S: Stuff happened that we couldn't live together, so I had to go stay with his [Randy's] mom again with Tyler [for five months].

I: Do you want to tell me more about that?

S: He [Randy] punched me in the face. And he got arrested, so it happened a lot. So the first time the cops were called and then that's when CAS [Children's Aid Services] got involved because they get involved when there's domestic violence and there's a kid in the house. So they were called, they came, and we were supposed to be getting counselling, and then one day he hit me really bad when I was holding Tyler. So I left, to stay with his mom ... His whole family knew that he had hit me but, you know, they were still his family ... so they were kind of like justifying what he did. So I went to Ontario [to Sarah's mother] for a month and then when I came back I went to live with Randy.

I: Did you take Tyler?

S: Yeah. Oh yeah, I don't leave him for more than a day. And so I came back from Ontario and then he hit me again and I called the police and he got arrested ... But the next day he came back ... and then there was a knock at the door and it was Ruth and that's my CP [child-protection] worker, and I opened the door and she came in and she said, "You have one of two choices. You can either stay here and I'll take Tyler or you can pack your stuff and leave right now ..."

Clearly, Sarah had a very strong attachment to her son as she agreed to leave her partner, but only if she could keep her son: "When it comes to Tyler—Randy will never win. My son will come first before anybody." Mirroring cases reported in other studies (Karabanow & Hughes, 2013), Sarah's relationship with her son superseded that with her partner. Yet, while the mother's position was clear and unwavering, David and colleagues (2012) argue that little is known about the specific influence of maternal psychological resilience (e.g., mother–child personality constructs, maternal problem-solving skills, and levels of maternal ego development) and ways it could buffer the impact of homelessness on her child.

In addition, Sarah took a risk to trust the support offered by her worker and move into supportive housing, as long as she could keep her son. Once there, she realized that her worker was trying to help as supportive housing provided stability and access to desired resources. As a result, the move fostered Sarah's determination to be a good mother.

S: When it [supportive housing] says ... supportive ... they are really supportive in what you want to do.

I: What's the high point for you—what's been the best thing?

S: Having Tyler, and [if it hadn't been for Tyler] then I wouldn't be here [supportive housing]. I'd probably still be bouncing everywhere.

During our second interview, Sarah remained firmly convinced that her move to supportive housing was a positive decision in that it provided structure, an organized physical environment, and access to material resources, programs, and support. While other mothers often complained about the rules and policies, by the second visit Sarah had enrolled in school, completed some courses, and received an academic achievement award for math. Similar to other studies reporting a strong motivation among homeless mothers to enhance their child's circumstances (Holtrop, McNeil, & McWey, 2015; Karabanow & Hughes, 2013; Narayan, 2015), Sarah was clear that having a child had been a turning point in her life that provided her with a new priority: she was determined to be a role model for her child. Indeed, a systematic literature review by Holtrop and colleagues (2015) found that many parents experiencing homelessness display positive outcomes, including those that are personal (cope effectively, meet basic family needs, experience reduced psychopathology); dyadic (demonstrate positive parenting practices and promote child adjustment); and contextual (exit episodes of homelessness and avoid shelter re-entry).

I: What makes you motivated?

S: Well, I want Tyler to be a high person in society. I don't want him to be a bum. And I don't want him to be on welfare … and yeah … I can't very well tell him to go finish school and go some place with his life if I haven't done it myself.

Sarah also had reconnected with Randy and both had begun abuse counselling in an effort to meet child protection's requirements to re-engage as a family. She explained, "We've been doing programs and doing what we've got to do … I go every two weeks and he goes every two weeks, and we just … talk about Tyler." Over time, child protection gained confidence in Sarah's parenting skills to the point where monitoring visits became a "fun chat":

I see her [child protection worker] maybe once a month for like ten minutes. Like she says, "Hi, what's up, what's Randy doing? Is he still going to program, you going to program?" … She doesn't come in my house, she don't need to see Tyler. She don't look him up and down for bruises. She don't look in my fridge. She comes in and says hi, hi, bye, bye. So it's not like I mind it, but even still, if I had someone over or something when she comes, it's like, who's that person? … Oh, nobody. Cuz it's embarrassing, right?

At the same time, a critical observation noted by Sarah, and other mothers in our study, was that child protection was the ever-present watchful eye—even if their parenting was not in question.

> I was never really embarrassed about CAS because it wasn't a parenting problem with me. It was like a domestic problem, I guess you call it. And my CAS worker told me, we had absolutely no concerns about your parenting at all and that I'm a better parent than a lot of the forty-year-olds they see. And even I have a home visitor from Family Resource Centre and she told me that she finds too a lot of people see the young moms sometime, well most time, are like, she didn't really say better than older moms just because … I'm not trying to prove nothing. I know I'm a good mom. I do everything for my kid.

By the third interview, given that both Sarah and Randy had completed their CAS programs successfully, Sarah noted that the highlight of the last several months was that child protection had closed their case. The family was getting together regularly and both parents were focused on enhancing their parenting skills. At the same time, despite her interest in moving back in with Randy, Sarah was reluctant to leave supportive housing until her allowable term (two years) was complete:

> No, I don't wanna leave … I don't even mind the rules, because most of the rules would be rules that I would have if I lived on my own anyway. And I like having the rules because if my friends, or something, say, "Oh Sarah, can I come stay the night?" … I don't like people staying the night, and I can just say, "No, nobody's allowed to stay."

In addition, Sarah had very clear expectations of Randy if they were to remain a couple:

> He's starting school in September. But I told him he has to start school—well, he doesn't have to, he has a choice, he can either start school in September or say goodbye. Because I'm not working my ass off to get a good job and go to

school and then him just sit around on welfare and do nothing. And 'cause, I want to show [Randy] that, you know, go to fucking school … I don't think he wants to go to school but I think he will. I just don't know how dedicated he'll be in school. But he needs to do something 'cause his mom's been on welfare for ten years and pretty much coaches him into staying on welfare and milking everything you can get out of them … I'm really embarrassed about being on welfare; my parents were never on welfare.

Despite Sarah's conviction to do everything possible to ensure that she provides a positive life for her son, her trajectory also highlighted her vulnerability in trying to control all challenges. When a city-wide transit strike threatened her ability to get to school and Tyler's daycare, Sarah once again recognized the critical role that supportive housing could play, and asked for help.

I was almost losing my daycare spot [due to the transit strike], because I have subsidy, right? And with subsidy, your kid is only allowed to miss like eight days in a month. So I was missing all this; I couldn't bring him to daycare, but there was a girl that came here [supportive housing] … she volunteers here or something, and she volunteered, twice a week to bring kids to daycare, like drive us to drop them off and stuff. So that was cool. But I was so scared I was gonna lose my spot.

Sarah had also gained enough confidence to seek out other community resources, which, as other studies have found (Campbell-Grossman, Hudson, Keating-Lefler, & Heusinkvelt, 2009; Campbell-Grossman et al., 2009), provide a comfortable venue to make friends and gain social support. In particular, these resources provide four different types of social support: informational (facts and knowledge), appraisal (affirmation and feedback), emotional (trust and esteem), and tangible (material resources) (Campbell-Grossman et al., 2009, p. 242).

I went with the Family Resource Centre and I love [it]! So, I love all their programs and I love all their staff … they're groups, right? So, it's like a lot of social, you get to talk with other moms … but pretty much everything they said I kind of already knew. Like I've been a mom for a while, so I get it.

Clearly, others thought she had made great progress as well, as Sarah had been asked by the supportive housing staff to give a speech at a fundraising event.

By the final interview, it was obvious that Sarah had made significant progress in a number of ways. Sarah's mother had visited and taken her camping, where she had been able to reconcile with her sister. She also had started volunteering at the adult psychiatric hospital to build her resumé for her college application. In addition, Randy had started school and his mother was now helping with childcare. Sarah was very positive in her reflection, noting a number of markers of stability, including food, housing, social support, and meaningful activity:

> **S:** It's [life is] much better now … Well, I don't got to worry where I'm sleeping. I got a bed. Yes, and I always have milk now. What's better, we always have food, which is better. I made friends. I definitely have more friends now than I did then [a year ago]. So that I know that if I ever did go in that situation I'd probably have more help than I did then. 'Cause all I had then was [Randy's] mom and his family.
>
> **I:** So what in your life now makes you feel happy and healthy?
>
> **S:** Tyler, Tyler's dad, my friends, my school, and my volunteering.

In addition, Sarah had a solid cluster of resources:

> **S:** I go to the [name] Family Resource Centre … I have a home visitor and she just talks to me about stuff … And my mom helps me. My mom sends me money … I do use the food bank once in a while. It comes here every Wednesday, so we get stuff. Well, Youth Employment Project, they support me in my schooling and stuff.
>
> **I:** So what has made it possible to get where you are now to succeed?
>
> **S:** Supportive housing, Tyler, welfare's definitely helped. I just don't—I don't like being on it … got to do what you got to do.

Sarah also was clear about what would keep her stably housed in the future: "I'm going to school to get a job … Well, I can't stay on welfare and expect him to finish school if I don't finish school …" At the end of the interview cycle, Sarah continued to reiterate that the birth of her son was the turning point in her life. For that reason, the fact that Sarah's greatest worry—that she would lose her child—had been reduced was perhaps one of the most important markers of her progress:

> S: [I worried before] that children's services would take my kid 'cause I wasn't stable and stuff. That's all I ever worry about 'cause everything I do, I do for him.

> I: Is there anything about yourself that you think has gotten you where you are now?

> S: I'm more motivated now that I have [Tyler] … than I was before I had [Tyler]. I just didn't care then, but now if I mess up my life, I mess up his life too, which is a sin …

> I: As you think about the past year, what has been positive?

> S: A lot of things. Like getting back to school, definitely positive. I don't drink, that's positive. I have a place to live. I don't know, things are just more certain now. Like I know that I have a home to come to. I know my kid has diapers and stuff … It's definitely harder work. It's easier to sit down and do nothing … Yes, I definitely do [like it better].

Sarah's experiences reflect her self-reported mental well-being scores (quality of life, mental health, and hope), which, while generally higher than those of Stephanie, Marcus, and Dean, did not shift significantly throughout the year (see Figure 1). In addition, Sarah's comments help to illustrate a theme common to the sample as a whole. Despite housing and homelessness being a key factor in young people's experiences that must be addressed, it was often progress and transitions in other areas of young people's lives that were particularly meaningful to them and that had a special impact on their future. Successes identified by other youth in the sample included finally being free of any criminal charges or criminal justice conditions, being able to meaningfully address addictions and mental health concerns, finding employment, and reconnecting with estranged family members. This theme reminds us that when designing interventions to address homelessness, we must ensure that youth are receiving the supports they need to address these other important aspects of life and that supporting these other successes is a key aspect of young people maintaining their housing.

CONCLUSION

The aim of this chapter was to better understand the process outlined in Chapter 2 using case studies to illustrate the distinct pathways of each subgroup. One particular observation was the significant levelling nature of the numerous challenges experienced by homeless youth that focused on broad *systematic* and *situational* barriers, while challenges such as race, ethnicity, and other significant demographics seemed to be less prominent in narratives. In particular, many youth had little knowledge of, and/or poor access to, supports and resources. And even when resources were available, system policies and procedures often dominated interactions, resulting in staff merely managing rather than truly assisting youth. Hudson and colleagues (2008) had similar findings and also identified four interpersonal barriers to care from service providers: authoritative communication, one-way communication, disrespect, and lack of empathy.

On the other hand, youth in our study who found stable housing and began to move forward noted the critical role played by those staff who seized the moment, truly engaged with them, and worked collaboratively to find ways to meet youth-identified (rather than staff-identified) goals. Others (Hudson et al., 2008; Mayberry, 2016) also have found that positive service experiences include those that are tailored to user needs and marked by clear and consistent communication between both parties.

Another critical observation from the quantitative data of our study noted that youth, even those who began to move forward, continued to struggle greatly in terms of their mental well-being and community integration despite having attained housing. Such observations reflect the findings of other qualitative studies of youth early in the process of exiting the streets (Karabanow, 2008; Kidd & Davidson, 2007). In contrast with their initial hopes about what might happen after exiting homelessness, most young people in transition struggled for some time in their efforts to build a meaningful life away from the streets and to deal with the physical and mental health sequelae resulting from major adversity during their childhood and adolescence.

It was in the qualitative data that the full complexity of building lives after homelessness became evident. While the one-year study period did not provide sufficient time to fully capture the trajectories that generally unfold over much longer periods, we did capture, across youth narratives, three major stages occurring along these longer trajectories. The first stage, an *initial turning point*, emerged as a tenuous hold on some form of housing stability, alongside continually high levels of adversity and connection with street activities. This stage reflects earlier work with youth contemplating exiting homelessness (Karabanow, 2008; Kidd & Davidson, 2007). Despite some engagement of supports and movement towards stability during this stage, youth faced barriers at the individual level (e.g., addictions, continued engagement with street social networks and activities) and structurally (e.g., challenges obtaining benefits and identification, and uncertainty about how to engage education and employment resources). In the second stage, *basic stability but limited forward momentum*, youth had obtained a basic level of stability and the risks of homelessness were less immediate. Despite this enhanced stability, young people in this stage felt stalled in their ability to achieve larger life goals. In the third stage, *looking to the future and beginning to achieve broader life goals*, youth were experiencing some tangible successes with these life goals. At this point, a hope-generating momentum became evident, although street-related challenges such as past criminal records, and the expense and difficulty of getting them expunged, continued to hamper progress. All three stages were similar for independent youth and mothers; however, pregnancy and childcare brought a flood of additional responsibilities.

At the individual level, however, the diversity of pathways becomes clearer—albeit qualified by the relatively small amount of time we had to understand them. Similar to Stephanie's ratings, exiting homelessness can be a much more challenging and drawn-out process than youth anticipate. Even though Marcus gained more stability than Dean, Stephanie began to meet some critical goals, and Sarah made a number of critically positive changes in her life, their ratings regarding future, quality of life, and mental well-being did not change dramatically. It may be that the effects of early life trauma continued. Reviewing Sarah's views over time, it is clear that while her ratings of quality of life and self-concept were fairly similar to those of the participant group as a whole, she experienced greater hope and community integration than most participants. In terms of community integration, while Sarah's views fluctuated over the year, by visits three and four they had stabilized at a fairly positive level. These ratings are consistent with her positive beliefs about the contribution of supportive housing. Similarly, while Sarah's initial feelings of hope were high, and dropped significantly by visits two and three, they were higher by visit four—consistent with her accomplishments over the year and realistic plans for the future. And while Sarah's ratings reflect some positive attributes, it is important to note that her ratings were not all positive and they definitely did not reflect the norm (see Figure 1).

Overall, we found that, with a fair degree of uniformity, the young people we studied are generally not flourishing, despite their having obtained stable housing. This may reflect service sectors that emphasize crisis response rather than health promotion or prevention (Altena, Brilleslijper-Kater, & Wolf, 2010; Slesnick et al., 2009), leaving few resources available to support youth after they have accomplished the challenging task of finding housing. It is clear that greater attention must be focused on what post-homelessness supports these young people require in order to build a mainstream life. For a mother, this task involves simultaneously rebuilding her own life, while building a life for her child. Hence, declining hope may well reflect not only the false promises that attend housed life, but also entry into a sphere in which many believe that they do not belong and cannot make gains. This is particularly worrisome given the extremely high suicide risk among this population, and the risks of returning to homelessness and addictions (Roy et al., 2009, 2014).

Mental health issues resonated through all these stages and trajectories. These issues had many causes, including exposure to adversity and violence before being on the streets, experiences of trauma and victimization while homeless, and the isolation and disappointment associated with exiting homelessness. For many, transforming their identity and lifestyle and improving their well-being required addressing mental health challenges resulting from traumatic experiences, and developing the ability to trust other people. For mothers, this meant developing trust in service providers, particularly those associated with child protection— despite fears of losing their child—in the hopes of building a stable family. Dealing with these challenges, and focusing on the positive features of their new way of life, despite systemic barriers that seem designed to undo their efforts, is a tremendous challenge greatly eased by external supports. Clearly, Sarah took a great risk in deciding to put her trust in one particular CAS staff who not only acknowledged Sarah's dilemmas (e.g., whether to leave her boyfriend or give up her baby), but also continued to work collaboratively throughout the year with her identified goals. While terrified of her CAS worker in her first interview, by the final visits Sarah fully recognized and trusted the continued support provided by her worker.

With respect to practice implications, as others have commented (Altena et al., 2010; Kidd, 2012; Slesnick et al., 2009), there is a pressing need for enhanced interventions for homeless youth, ones that carefully evaluate the complex traumatic experiences of youth and create targeted interventions (Wong, Clark, & Marlotte, 2016) with evidence to support best-practice models. This is true for all youth who have exited the streets, but particularly for mothers (Campbell-Grossman, Brage Hudson, Keating-Lefler, & Ofe Fleck, 2005; Campbell-Grossman et al., 2009; Schrag & Schmidt-Tieszen, 2014). The resources available to youth who successfully exit the streets are inadequate due to a systemic emphasis on crisis-oriented services and criminalization in social response. Young people who have transitioned out of homelessness have demonstrated tremendous resilience in obtaining housing instead of becoming chronically homeless into adulthood, being jailed for lengthy periods, or losing their lives. Once housed, most struggled greatly for protracted periods, seeking to establish a stable existence. Our work suggests that supported housing and community workers can assist in this process. What is most needed is a set of integrated supports and services that address both the structural challenges (employment opportunities) and subjective components (such as quality of life) associated with these transitions. Also needed are care providers who not only understand the developmental needs and histories of homeless youth, but also have the skills to take strengths-based approaches to work collaboratively with youth-identified needs. We predict that economic analysis of such an approach will readily demonstrate considerable monetary savings as more youth become contributing members of communities and society at large, rather than continuing to have costly interactions with social services and the criminal justice system over the long term.

CHAPTER 4

The Wickedness of Youth Homelessness ... Our Knowledge Mobilization Process

Taking a step back from the specific findings of our study, it can be seen that youth homelessness is a field of study across research, practice, and policy that can be considered a "wicked" problem. A wicked problem is one that is not amenable to a purely scientific or rational approach, suffers from unclear problem definition, is interdependent with other social problems, and is variably viewed depending on the stakeholder perspective. The wicked nature of this social problem is readily attested to in its persistence over time and across widely diverse contexts, and in the consistent failure to generate research that can be translated into real-world impacts. As such, the complexity and subtleties of this phenomenon, in terms of its social, psychological, economic, and political dimensions, makes for research that is primarily micro in scope, and incomplete and partial in analysis. Substantive change seems to require large-scale sociopolitical movements, which make use of information provided by researchers to varying degrees, if at all. In the area of both youth and adult homelessness, examples of such movements include the work of the Social Reformers in the late nineteenth century, Roosevelt's New Deal initiative in the 1930s, and, potentially, the international housing first initiatives in recent years (Kidd, 2004; Kidd & Taub, 2004). Systemic problems clearly require systemic solutions. Unfortunately, most homeless research is only loosely connected to the systems relevant to youth homelessness.

We grappled with this situation in our own work. We had successfully completed a complicated two-site study examining pathways towards stability; had a large amount of data, which has been laid out in the previous chapters; and were not content to publish only in peer-reviewed journals accessed almost exclusively by a small group of elite and enfranchised academics and their students. We wanted to share what we found with the communities involved and, most importantly, wanted to reach individuals in government who have the power to change policies and set agendas in a manner that can have systemic impacts. We recognized that such individuals have projects and ideas pitched to them continually, are grappling with extremely demanding workloads and often dispersed responsibilities, and set strategy within a finite time period—typically their term in office. These individuals are seldom researchers and service providers, and they may not have a particular interest in homeless youth. Given these assumptions, we questioned what our communication strategy should be.

One idea that we rejected was hosting a standard "knowledge translation" (KT) event. By this we mean an afternoon or day, usually catered and in a nice setting, where researchers use PowerPoint to present a study and its findings; potentially facilitate round-table discussions about relevant issues, problems, and solutions; and reconvene as a large group at the end to answer questions and likely provide a report. We recognized evidence-based challenges with this approach, mainly the fact that people do not learn well from, or do much following, PowerPoint presentations of information (Bannister & O'Sullivan, 2013; Buchko, Buchko, & Meyer, 2012). But frankly, we were mainly tired of delivering and attending this type of forum. Many people will turn up if you are connected via social networks. People will nod and smile, work on their smartphones, get caught up with one another's personal lives, and then take the report back to their office to be buried among a dozen similar, never-read documents, completely forgetting that the event ever happened unless directly reminded. This probably is a cynical view, but it is one that resonated with us. Such is the well-worn path of most KT efforts in academia.

Our group wanted to break away from this tedious format, with its limited impacts. Returning to basic principles of how information can have an impact, we recognized that any effort to make a difference in the lives of people like our participants (a cause to which we are passionately committed) needs a better approach. Fundamentally, we wanted to sell the idea that unless we improve supports for young people who are leaving homelessness, we are wasting resources, opportunities, and, ultimately, lives. Taking a cue from people in advertising and business, who are superb at selling ideas, we considered the characteristics of effective communication put forward by Heath and Heath (2008):

1. The message is simple.
2. There is an element that is unexpected.
3. Suggestions are concrete.
4. The source is credible.
5. It draws upon and cultivates an emotional response.
6. It shares information through stories.

There is a large body of evidence to suggest that marketing campaigns—whether selling soap, airplane rides, or activism—are more successful if they do these six things. Given that our research involves people, rather than products, we felt that there were ethical imperatives that must also be met if communication of our research is to be considered successful. We therefore set ourselves three further standards for an effective message:

7. It is true to the experiences of our participants.
8. It is deeply respectful of their experiences.
9. They are involved in its creation.

We began an intensive process to consider how we might do a good job of addressing these nine points—work that we did with our service provider partners and those research participants who wanted to be involved in advocacy. Tackling items one and three was mostly a task of overcoming our academic inclinations. Academics, mired in complexities like intersectional frameworks of marginalization, are usually very poor at generating simple messages. Item three was a bit easier since several of us have worked as service providers, so we had some skill at translating findings into concrete suggestions. We could fairly easily come up with something clear and concrete along the lines of, "These youth need support or they will end up homeless again, and here are a few things that would make a difference: unconditional care, transition-oriented case management, peer support, education/meaningful activity, building acceptance and belonging, and addressing mental health and wellness."

Items four and seven to nine were not very difficult for our group. Across academic, service provider, and lived-experience domains we have collective credibility, and our meaningful engagement of youth in advocacy efforts aligns with the final three points. Moreover, we have diverse experiences with homeless youth with regards to research, service delivery, policy development, and knowledge translation/mobilization. Furthermore, we decided on a participatory framework for this component of the research because it provided us an opportunity to check on the validity of our findings, to generate additional insights and nuance about those findings, and to give our participants an opportunity to be at the table and to have a say in how their stories were shared and communicated (Conrad, 2004; Cornwall & Jewkes, 1995; Reason, 1998).

The major challenges were filling in the gaps, particularly aspects of the unexpected; enhancing emotional investment; and employing stories powerfully. These challenges seemed to us to have a fairly obvious answer: the arts. There is a certain amount of cliché around youth and art, perhaps embodying an assumption that all youth are invariably interested in, and involved with, the arts. Despite the cliché, we did believe from past experience that involvement in the arts can be impactful for those generating the art, and for others who engage with it (Karabanow & Naylor, 2015; Kidd, 2009). One of our principal investigators, Jeff Karabanow, had made a documentary film with young people on the streets in Guatemala City, as well as an art-filled book on youth homelessness, and, together with another of our investigators, Jean Hughes, created animated shorts with young people in Halifax, illustrating lived experiences of homelessness, street culture, marginalization, and notions of hope. These initiatives, despite their different cultural contexts, gave way to spaces of care, sanctuary, and critical consciousness, while the resulting art products continue to sensitize and educate segments of civil society (see Karabanow & Naylor, 2015). In addition, unlike the usual KT events, the arts-based products generated some action. For example, the Halifax-based animated video was posted on YouTube and advertised in the university news, resulting in the university dental clinic agreeing to change its practice and accept homeless people with emergency dental problems.

There is a large literature demonstrating the broad value of art in clinical and social service contexts (Star & Cox, 2008; Tesch & Hansen, 2013; Walsh, 2008; White, 2006; Windsor, 2005). Osei-Kofi (2013) notes that while arts-based research is not new, it's becoming increasingly popular because of its potential to "honor multiple ways of knowing, including sensory knowing" (p. 137). Furthermore, at the centre of arts-engaged research is the capacity to co-create knowledge with research participants, engage reflexively with the research process, and "embody great potential for consciousness raising and critical dialogue" (Osei-Kofi, 2013, p. 137). In this way, art in the context of a research project has the ability to do a number of important things: to capture and communicate different ways of knowing and nuanced elements of experience; to unite researchers and participants and to flatten power differentials; to create interpersonal connections and meaning in shared experience; to offer different ways through which to understand and critique oppressive social systems; and to create emotional resonance, understanding, and empathy on the part of the researchers, participants, and audience. The context provided by the creating and sharing of art also struck us as a fun, energizing, and warm environment in which to discuss and share the findings of our research.

Based on these past experiences, we organized a KT event with a twist. While we invited the usual suspects (academics, policy-makers, service providers), we tried to shake up the format somewhat by incorporating the arts in several ways:

1. We modelled the event after an art showing. We held it at an arts organization for marginalized youth, prominently displayed the art, and had the event catered by a social business (a catering company staffed by marginalized youth).
2. We held the event in the early evening, timed to not interfere with the workday but also to not be late enough that people would go home and change their minds about going.
3. We had several spoken word, poetry, and music performances by young people interspersed throughout the evening.

4. We briefly shared key study findings and made concrete suggestions for addressing the challenges we identified.
5. We thanked specific individuals for coming so they were identified and openly acknowledged.

One final arts-based strategy had the greatest impact. Knowing that the fate of most well-crafted reports is to be recycled or deleted, we opted to present our research findings in a novel form: a comic. The main focus of this chapter is the process of crafting this creative research report.

FIRST STEPS

There are many interesting examples of how arts generally, and animation and comics specifically, have been leveraged to engage with and draw attention to a range of wicked problems (Head, 2008). Though, as a group, we were aware of such efforts, and had been involved in some ourselves, the idea of a comic resulted specifically from one of our team members' prior knowledge of comic artist Sarafin's work, through her series *Asylum Squad*. We loved Sarafin's artistic style, wry sense of humour, and critical voice (Smith, 2010). Her approach to comic making felt like a good fit for our project. Our initial foray into the land of comics as KT resulted when, mid-project, we received a small bit of funding to share our preliminary findings with the public. We commissioned Sarafin, and another comic artist using a single-panel style, to develop comic artwork reflecting study themes:

In 2014, I had the joy and pleasure of working with a group of bright, talented young people on this comic ... it was a project designed to draw attention to some of the issues young people face when dealing with homelessness, and when trying to get off the streets. The group I worked with, consisting of Layla Sunshine, Baby T, and Orlando Foster, had all been homeless at one time or another themselves, as had I. Layla Sunshine, Baby T, and Orlando Foster wrote the comic, and I worked as the illustrator. In the end, we pulled together an honest, thought-provoking piece of work that gives insight into life on the streets, and the challenges one can face when trying to find a home ... I was recently asked while sitting on a panel at Massey College—why comics? My answer was that I felt that comics appeal to the inner child in all of us. Like little films on paper, they are accessible, both to make and to read. You don't need to spend too much money to make a comic book, and—unless it's some rare first-edition copy of a popular series—comics aren't too expensive to buy and enjoy either. It's no wonder that the film world so often turns to comics for inspiration—the two are cousins to one another. (Sarafin)

The idea was to give participants a short comic book they could take away with them, and to use the panels as a discussion point during the KT event. We had only a short time to get the book prepared, so for pragmatic reasons this pilot comic was strictly a commission, rather than a collaboration. We highlighted some key themes we wanted to get across, and Sarafin constructed a character and a narrative that communicated those themes. The result was a nine-page book called *Her Story*, which follows a young squeegee punk named Melanie from her initial turning point, when she was physically victimized on the street, through her struggles to find and maintain housing and then cut off old street friends, and eventually learning (spoiler alert!) that she is pregnant. The book turned out beautifully and was a huge hit at the event and among our community partners.

This initial success planted the seeds for a longer and more ambitious project that would allow us to tease out some of the complexity of our participants' lives, which were inevitably flattened to fit within a nine-page limit. With a little more lead time and a slightly larger budget (SSHRC graciously allowed us to reallocate our remaining funding), we returned to the comic idea, knowing that, in order to meet the ethical objectives we had set for ourselves for successful communication of our research findings, we must involve research participants in the construction of the comic. To accomplish this mission within a tight time frame, acknowledging the limitations of hand-selecting participants, we approached three respondents, each with a unique set of experiences. Although we had more time than with the first comic, time was still a factor, so we pragmatically chose participants we felt would be engaged and reliable and who would work well together. We acknowledge the limitations in hand-selecting participants this way, and recognize the obvious value in finding ways to include a wider range of participants (this includes individuals who are generally overlooked for these kinds of opportunities due to personal characteristics or struggles that might make it challenging to incorporate them in structured activities).

THE PROCESS OF DEVELOPMENT

The comic development process engaged participants in a series of meetings where, in collaboration with Sarafin, they developed the characters, plot, and storyline. Having never done this before, and with little guidance available from the academic literature, we hoped to be able to complete this process in three or four meetings. In the end it took five. Our goal was to have the participants incorporate a few key themes that we wanted to highlight about the process of exiting homelessness, while also incorporating issues and experiences from their own lives. We hoped that this synthesis would lend the comic an important depth and truthfulness, and ensure that it was both honest and respectful (again, see the standards for an effective message, items 7 to 9, above). After completing the comic, we reflected on the process and conducted debriefing interviews with the participants. In the next section we describe the successes of the project, as well as challenges faced and lessons learned. From these observations we make some recommendations designed to help guide researchers or practitioners who might be interested in trying something similar.

Engaging Participants

As noted above, it was important for us to structure this as a participatory project and to engage the participants from the research in the process. This approach created significant value for the comic, as well as for the participants helping us craft the comic. This section will discuss each set of outcomes in turn.

From the perspective of the story, involving the participants in the writing of the comic was particularly valuable because of their insights in crafting the language and for capturing some of the subtler nuance in interaction and experience. For example, there was a lot of discussion within the group about the section of the comic where the main character, Brandon, is at an emergency shelter and being asked for cigarettes by another youth. This is a small section within the comic as a whole, but there is a lot of important information wrapped in that interaction: the constant risk of exploitation in the shelter system, the direct and demanding way that youth can interact with each other in those settings, and the manipulation that happens through a complicated mix of intimidation and caring (i.e., demanding cigarettes but then offering advice and a kind word). Similarly, there was interesting discussion about the scene at the end when Brandon is interacting with his family. Based on our coding of the data, the research team was trying to highlight the desire of many of the youth in the sample for reconnection and the role it played in the exiting process. However, in crafting the scene, the writers of the comic introduced important themes of rejection, trust, feeling like a disappointment, and the never-ending work of having to manage strained family relationships. In retrospect, these themes were present throughout the interviews but never made it fully to the surface of our analytic framework. The participants in the comic were able to pull important and resonant themes from their own experience and to find a way to embed them in the story. From the perspective of the story, this was valuable because it served as a check on the validity of the data and also got us a little closer to an honest rendering of experience. It also deepened the analysis and helped communicate subtle and complicated themes about how the exiting process is experienced.

The participatory process also generated a lot of value in terms of allowing the writers of the comic to share their experience and tell their story. Certainly one of the most enjoyable parts of the comic creation process was witnessing those moments when the participants would swap stories around a particular theme—jumping in excitedly, and cutting each other off as they "cracked up" telling stories about all the "ridiculous" issues that landlords have given them a hard time about, or how they managed to get out of a jam when the cops turned up to kick them out of the park or to break up a party. The participants also commented on the value of these interactions, noting that it was nice to be able to tell stories and discuss their experiences with people who had been through something similar, particularly because they did not feel judged by people who shared similar experiences. These comments reinforced our general finding that a central issue facing young people as they exit from homelessness is figuring out where they fit in mainstream society, and managing the feeling that they are on the outside looking in—that society does not care about or even see them, rendering them invisible.

The comic development process provided a context in which youth who were going through the struggles of exiting homelessness could connect and share. This feature alone made the project tremendously valuable. As a rule, young people can be reluctant to engage with group therapy or counselling, and we see comic making as a good way to attract individuals to a group setting and to facilitate the process. The collaborative nature of the project gave youth a chance to meet and develop friendships with other young people who could understand their experience, but who were also at a stage in which they were trying to make a change. This opportunity to build support from peers who have successfully transitioned away from homelessness is critical given our findings that youth in our sample often self-isolated and distanced themselves from old friendship networks to avoid getting drawn back into street life. In addition, arts spaces have a way of building a sense of community and belonging (Karabanow & Naylor, 2015). They can, at times, plant the seeds for deeper bonding and sharing based on common experiences—a way to build critical consciousness in terms of understanding one's own journey vis-à-vis others' experiences, and collectively work to craft plans for the future.

The participants also commented that there was a more general value in being able to tell the story of homeless youth through the medium of comics. We observed a strong desire among all our study participants to find meaning in their difficult experiences. The comic spoke to this desire, and participants commented that the comic development process did help them find some meaning; they were able to be a part of something that might make a difference by helping the public and policy-makers to better understand the experiences of homeless youth. This section will now turn to a discussion of some of the challenges in the engagement process and lessons learned.

CHALLENGES AND LESSONS LEARNED

Challenges Due to Instability

A central finding of the project as a whole, and during the comic development process specifically, is that the process of exiting homelessness is a cyclical one characterized by ongoing setbacks. As we have mentioned, a year is not a very long time. Despite selecting youth who achieved relatively high levels of stability during the year, the comic development participants were not immune to such setbacks during this process. Their challenges were representative of those experienced across the sample during the formal study period, including job loss, breakups, unemployment, trouble paying rent, landlord issues, loss of housing, and struggles with addiction. These events, in addition to being heartbreaking, reinforced the underlying message of the comic—that exiting homelessness is a long and difficult process. The experiences of the comic development participants also helped to underscore the fact that the continuing poverty typical of people who have experienced homelessness means that there may never be a specific day when youth feel that they are fully stable, that their housing is 100 percent secure, and that the exiting process is totally complete. As such, core themes of instability and fragility underscore all aspects of our project.

Challenges with Scheduling

For a number of reasons, scheduling was one of the central logistical challenges of the whole comic-making process. The ongoing instability described above meant that participants' lives often were chaotic, making it unlikely that they would attend all scheduled meetings. The instability also meant that participants' phones were often temporarily out of commission, or the number was changed. With no cellphone number at which to contact them, we were forced to rely on email, which many of our participants barely used (seemingly due to generational changes in the popularity of email, and limited Internet access). This meant that there could be long delays in hearing back from participants, which made it very difficult to coordinate five people's unstable and constantly shifting schedules. Eventually we began to use DoodlePoll, a free online scheduling website, which helped but could not fully address the issue.

The main consequence of these scheduling challenges was that most meetings were missing one or two people. This was frustrating for everyone, because the group was committed to constructing the comic collaboratively and by consensus. This commitment meant that a significant portion of each meeting was spent reviewing progress from the previous week to ensure that everyone felt included in decision making and that participants did not feel that their ideas were being changed in their absence. In light of this experience, recognizing that life is often unpredictable for participants, our recommendation would be to build routine into the initiative by scheduling meetings at regular intervals (e.g., every Tuesday from noon to two), to provide participants with a hard copy of the schedule at the first meeting, and to send regular reminders to all the contact points for each person.

Challenges with the Process

Collaborative writing is a challenging process. At the beginning of the comic's development, we toyed with a few different strategies to overcome potential difficulties. For example, we considered making each person responsible for one section of the comic, but rejected that idea because it posed obvious problems in terms of workflow and maintaining a consistent voice. In addition, we originally planned to have a professional comic instructor help facilitate the process during the first couple of meetings, but a last-minute health problem meant that could not happen. We rejected the option of having each participant create his or her own comic because we wanted a single story that was long enough to adequately incorporate the key themes of this project. In future projects we would consider allowing all youth to craft their own individual stories, perhaps engaging multiple illustrators or encouraging participants to draw their own stories.

Given the challenges of collaborative writing, we recommend outlining a clear structure and goals for each meeting, and for the process as a whole. In our naïveté we adopted a more casual approach, thinking that the group was small enough to maintain an adequate structure on its own. This lack of formality left room for joking and informal interaction, which was beneficial, but it also meant that progress could be slow and meetings a little chaotic. We believe there is a balance to be struck between an informal and formal structure. Participants commented that they liked the time to chat and hang out, but that the process might also have been more enjoyable if the meetings were more structured and efficient.

Challenges with Engagement

A key element of the process proposed here is to allow the participants to fully engage with the research findings. As noted above, doing so is valuable for the comic-writing process in that it builds a strong understanding of the material, therefore facilitating incorporation of key themes into the comic. This also serves as an opportunity to "member check" the data, and gives respondents an opportunity to reflect on the findings for their own benefit and understanding. In practice, our tight time frame meant that we allowed only a short time for this part of the process, where we identified key themes for brief reflection and discussion within the group. In retrospect, it would have been preferable to dedicate more time to presenting all the findings to allow time for ongoing digestion, processing, and reflection. It became apparent during the process that participants desired this deeper level of engagement when a couple of the respondents asked to see a research team member's study notes so that they could read more of the quotes and engage with them on their own terms.

Challenges Due to Timing

This point has already been touched on a couple of times in previous sections, but it bears highlighting. The comic development process requires time. We found that our short five-meeting time frame meant that the process was compressed. This created a number of challenges. More time was needed to recognize the natural processes that participants go through when working as a team. This would have allowed further opportunity to fully discuss the study findings with participants, to incorporate informal time just to chat and "goof around" without feeling pressured to stay on task, and to take adequate time for each stage (developing characters, plot, and storyline), so that we could comfortably work through a lucid process of development rather than jumping right in. This also would have allowed time for the critical process of reflective thinking to assist participants in deeper understanding of the findings. Based on our experience, we recommend around eight two-hour sessions—moving in process from setting parameters, to becoming connected as a group, to solidifying main themes/ ideas, and then to allowing some reflexive review of initial sketches and a beta version of the comic. Recognizing the need for flexibility and time for reflection and group debriefing in each session, we suggest an example of how the initiative might proceed: meeting one, outlining process; meeting two, reviewing research results; meetings three to six, identifying characters and building narratives; meetings seven and eight, refining and editing.

REACTIONS

As the previous discussion has illustrated, the comic proved to be a successful way of connecting the participants with others who had been through similar experiences, and for providing them with an outlet to share their insights and experiences. Beyond these positive outcomes, which were internal to the process, we found that the comic was tremendously successful as a form of "knowledge translation."

Following the launch, we received much positive feedback from stakeholder groups, including frontline social service staff, youth with lived experience of homelessness, and policy-makers. Social service staff were drawn to the comic book as a nuanced and heartfelt representation of the challenges they see every day, and it was something that they wanted to share with their colleagues and clients. The youth we heard from were excited to see an output that they could connect with, and that was more than some bland graph. They also indicated that they felt inspired to do their own artmaking and storytelling. The comic also proved to be an effective tool for engaging policy-makers: core findings were presented in an easy-to-understand manner, employing an accessible and articulate art form. Indeed, for policy-makers, the comic was unexpected, and helped direct their divided attention to our project and our message. A similar reaction was experienced by service providers regarding the animated shorts created by youth in the Halifax context.

A central strength of the comic, which was at the heart of all the positive reactions we received, was that it was humanizing and had emotional resonance. The use of a fictional character has the (ironic) effect of helping to communicate to the reader that there are real people behind the facts, figures, and themes we are presenting. Watching the main characters go through ups and downs helps to show the complicated ways that individual, social, and systemic forces intertwine to make exiting homelessness exceedingly difficult. This effect is important because garnering support for long-term solutions to youth homelessness from policy-makers and the public depends on those groups appreciating the way that societal inaction stifles the potential of so many vibrant young people, and the real human suffering that is so commonplace.

A final benefit to using a comic as KT is that, as a work of craft and art, it is much harder to throw away than a conventional handout or a report. It is probably safe to assume that most materials shared at KT events barely make it past the first recycling bin! The advantage of a comic is that it is a conversation piece that people can put on their desk or coffee table and show to their friends and colleagues, which helps to broaden the reach of an event beyond its immediate time and place!

CONCLUSION

One of our objectives for this study was to develop a meaningful and creative narrative communicating the experiences of young people exiting the street, and finding and maintaining stable housing. In doing so, we wished to use a popular art medium as a form of graphic knowledge mobilization that could provide a *springboard to action* for decision makers, policy-makers, service providers, and educators—particularly in the frame of wicked problem contexts from which the often linear and circumscribed frames of traditional research can seem detached and ineffective. One unintended consequence of this work was that it helped to create a space where some of our research participants were able to openly share their stories of trauma, failure, fragility, and broken dreams, and also of hope, laughter, new dreams, and life. In the small art studio where our comic was created, there was a sense of belonging and connection. Comic work produced in such a fashion assumes an audience in a way that an interview or survey does not, and has the ability to convey emotion and engender empathy in audiences. The following chapter showcases the comic book and, as such, makes sense of a complex phenomenon through an engaging visual narrative format driven by some of our youth participants.

CHAPTER 5

A Long Way to Go

ABOUT THE PROJECT

This comic was conceived as a way to communicate the findings of a SSHRC-funded research project that followed fifty-one young people from Halifax and Toronto over the course of a year as they made efforts to transition away from homelessness. A comic seemed like a perfect way to highlight key themes, and also as a way to draw attention to the real people and the real stories behind this issue. Right now there are young people out there, like the character in the book, who are doing everything they can to get out of the trap that homelessness creates—a journey characterized by setbacks and major systemic barriers, but also helping hands and incredible strength and resilience. We also hope that the comic will serve as a call to action that collectively we must do everything we can to support formerly homeless young people as they work towards stability and their personal, educational, and career goals. As the comic illustrates, the stakes are too high not to.

The comic book was created from start to finish by three incredible young people who participated in the research project, along with the amazing comic artist Sarafin (Sarah Griffin). Drawing from findings from the research, along with their own personal experiences, they created the characters, the story, and the dialogue. All of us involved with the project couldn't be more excited and proud of what they created. We would like to specifically thank all of the youth that participated in the research who shared their insights, time, and experiences with us and who made the project such a success. We would also like to thank SSRHC and the CAMH Foundation for their financial support, and our community partners in Halifax and Toronto for their immeasurable help with the research and the continuing work they do to support young people. A special thanks to Ark (Halifax), SHYM (Halifax), LOFT Community Services (Toronto), Covenant House (Toronto), and SKETCH (Toronto). The research team includes Sean Kidd (PI), Jeff Karabanow (PI), Jean Hughes, Ted Naylor, Tyler Frederick, Michal Chwalek, Andrea Reynolds, Marianne Quirouette, Kait Sullivan, Kelly Fenn, and Caila Aube.

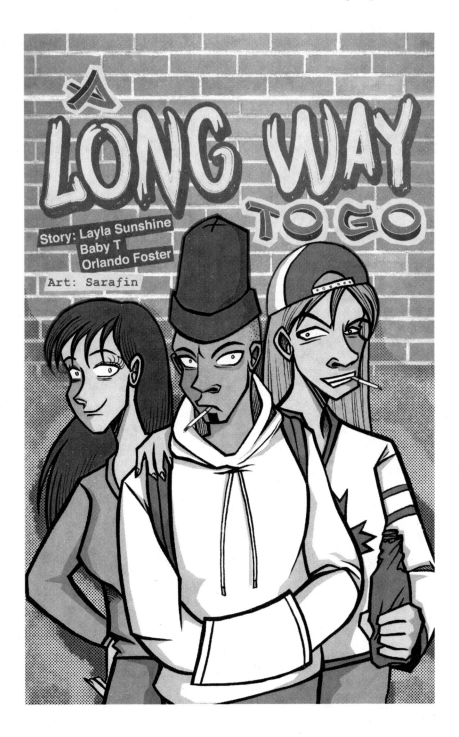

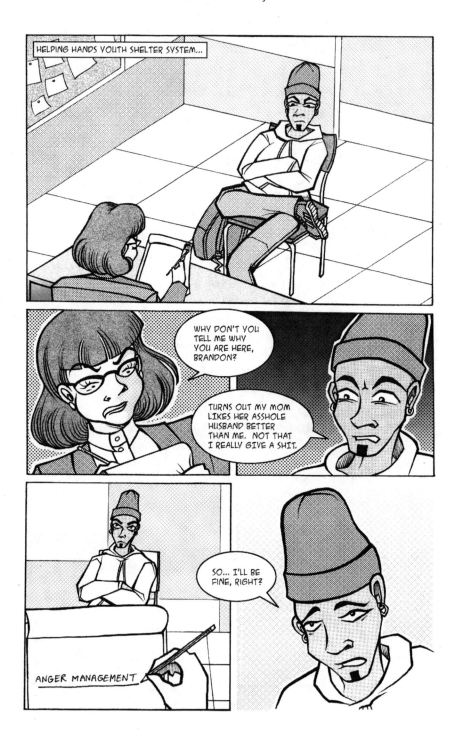

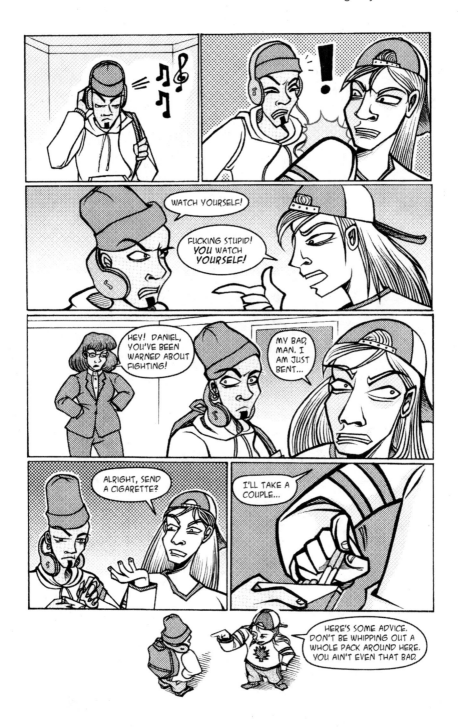

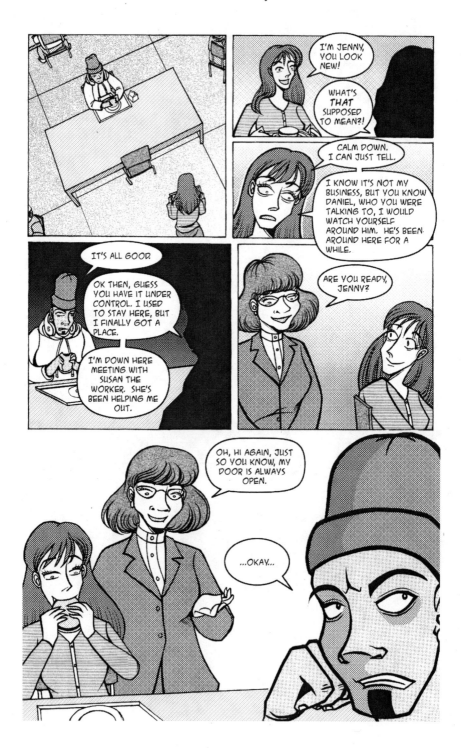

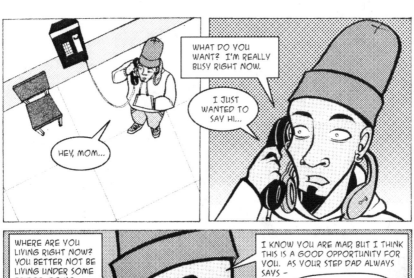

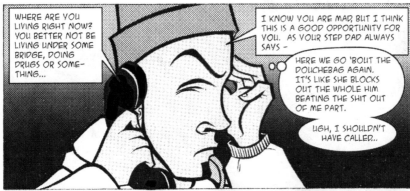

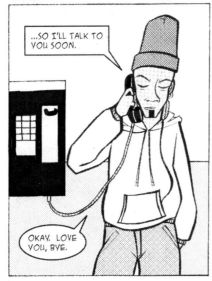

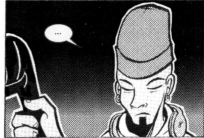

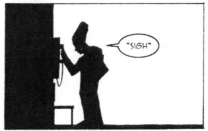

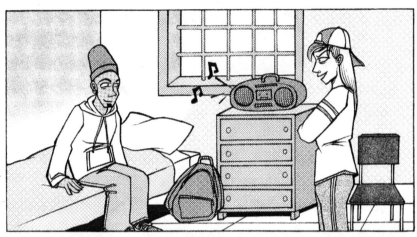

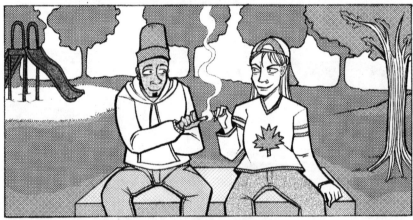

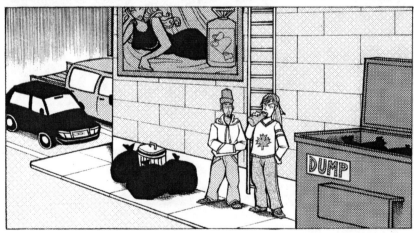

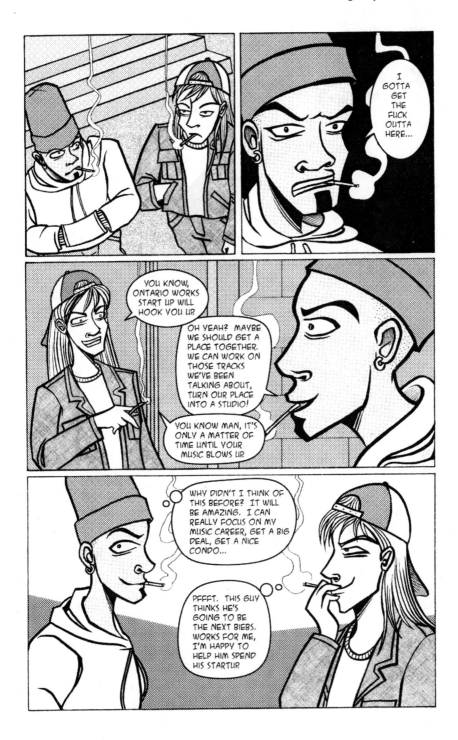

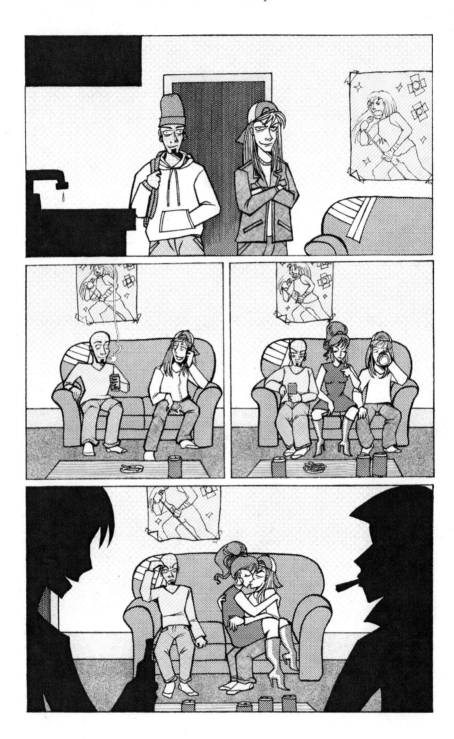

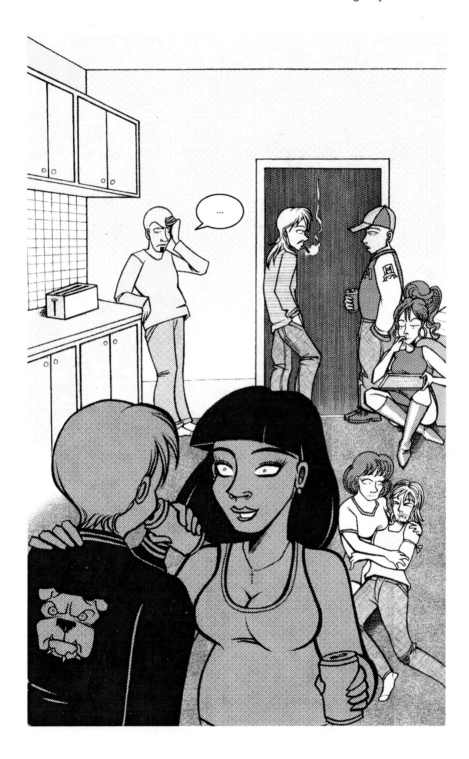

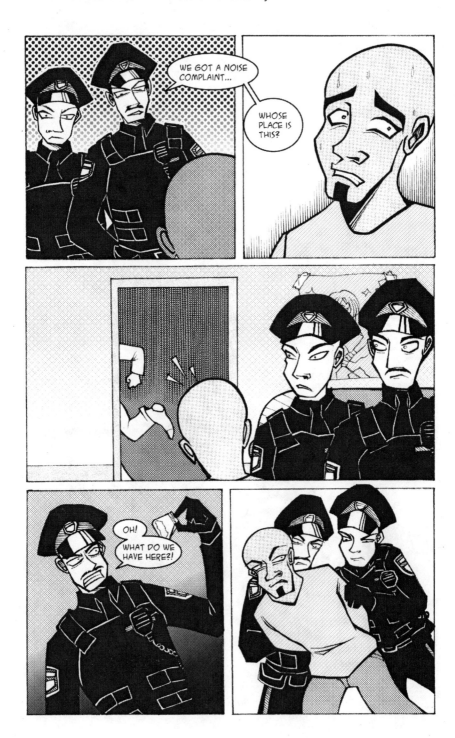

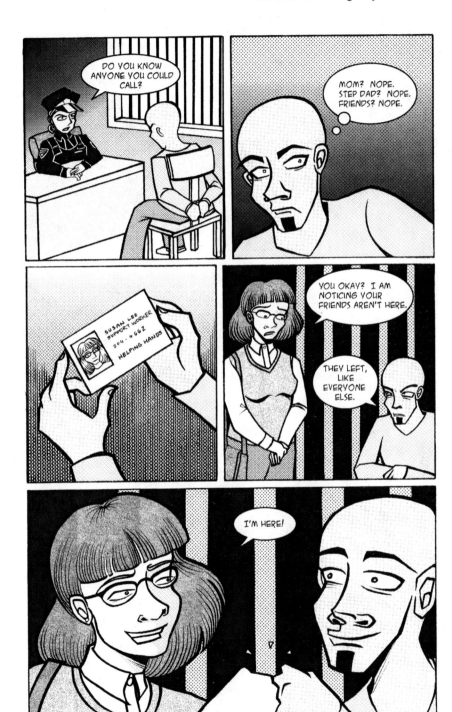

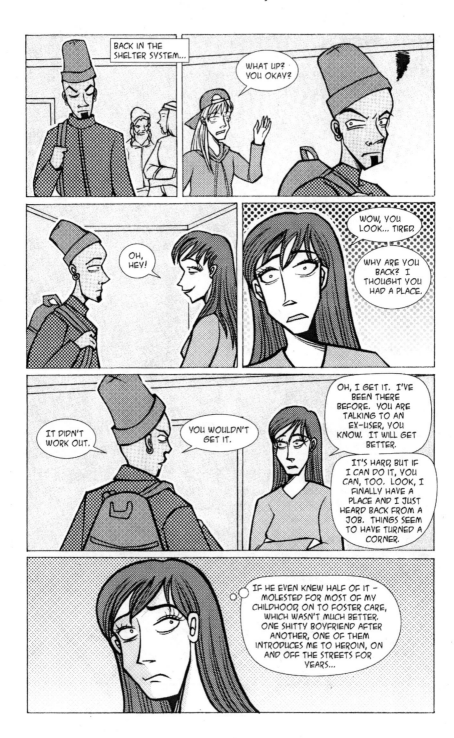

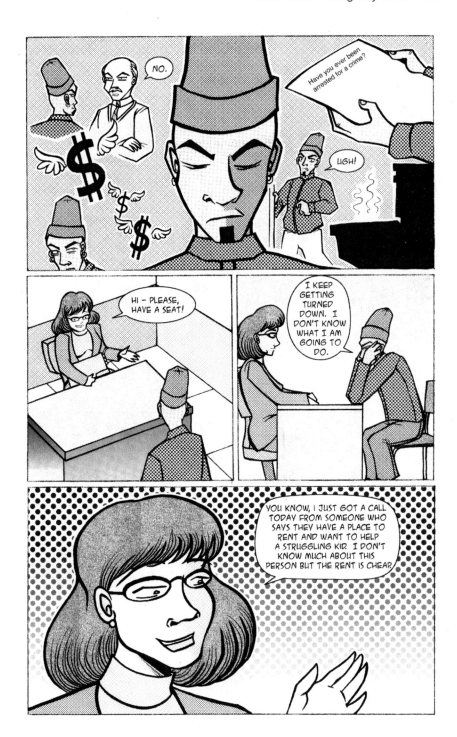

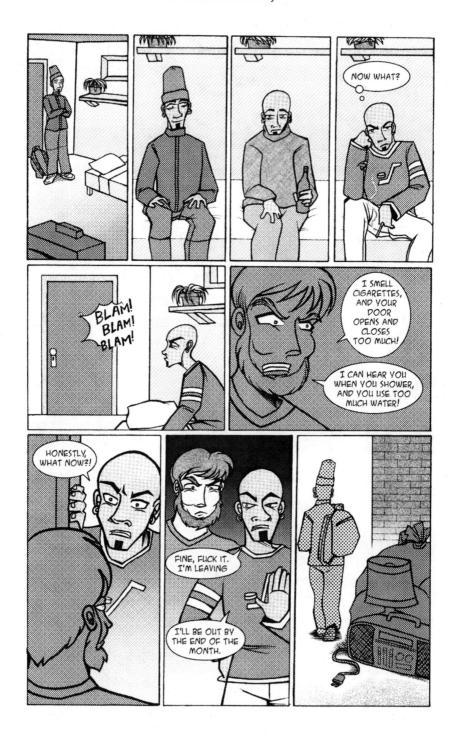

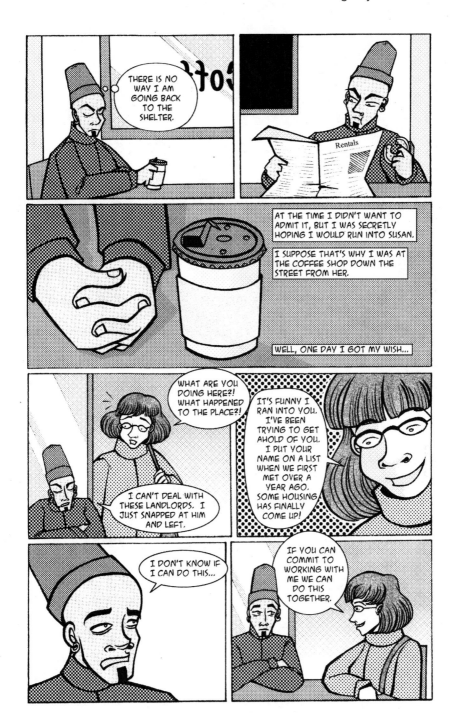

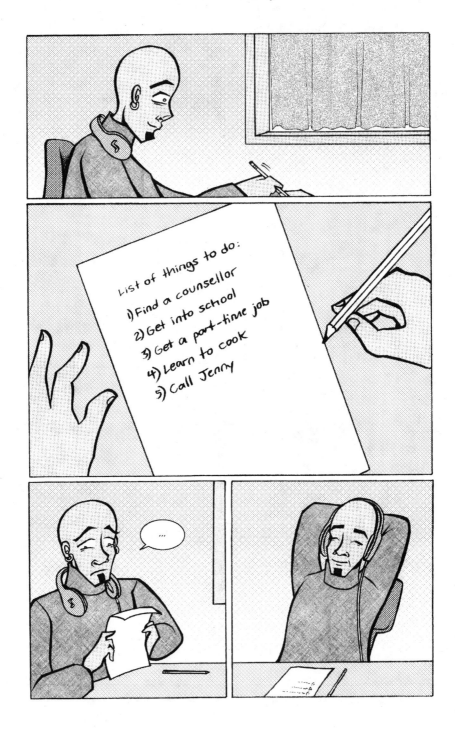

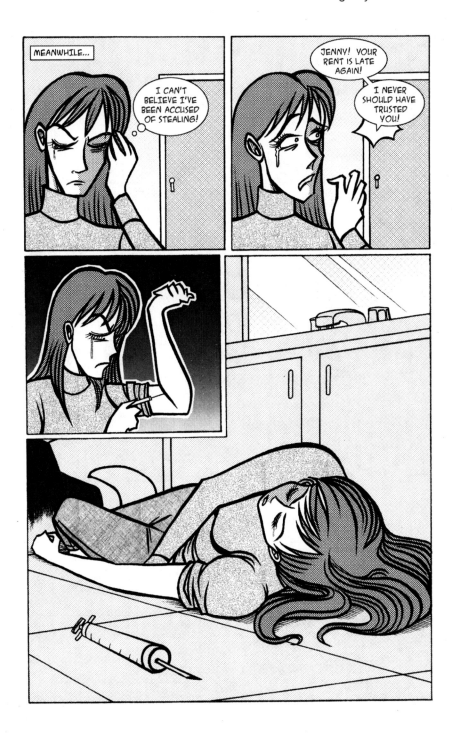

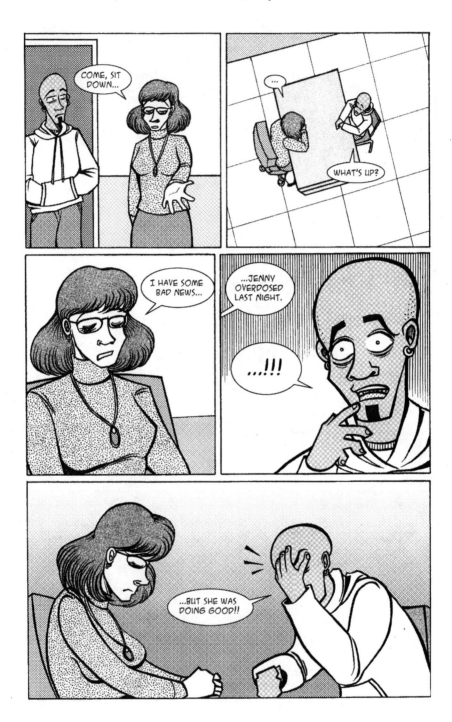

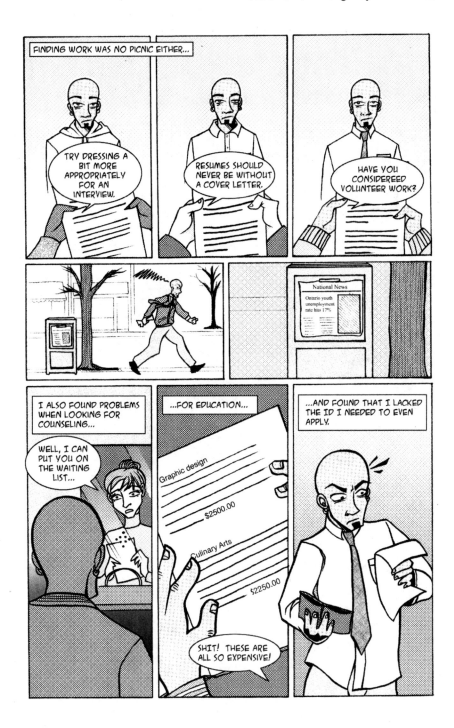

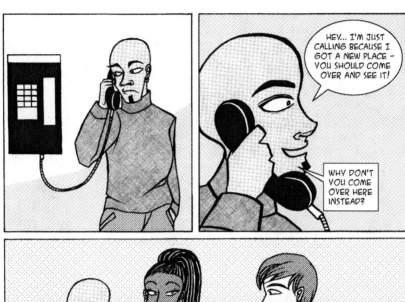

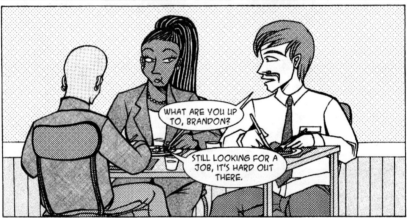

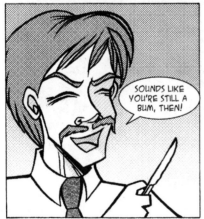

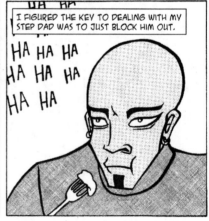

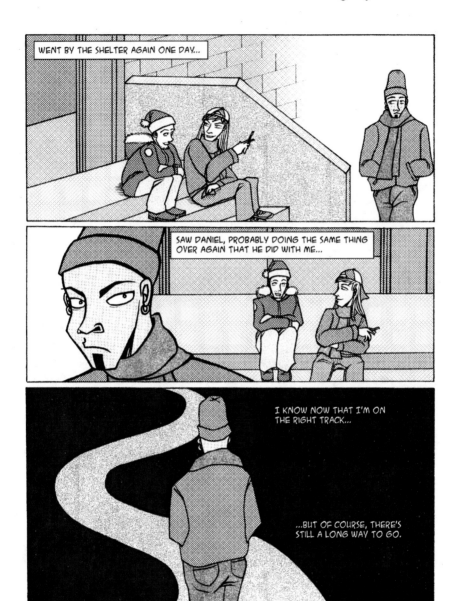

THESE STORIES AND STORIES LIKE
THEM ARE HAPPENING EVERY DAY
ALL TOO OFTEN STEPS OUT OF
HOMELESSNESS MEET
INSURMOUNTABLE BARRIERS AND
A RETURN TO THE STREETS, TO
HOSPITALS, TO PRISONS

We can make a difference by:
- **Providing decent housing**
- **Providing supports during and after the transition from the streets – supports that don't end when youth turn 25**
- **Addressing mental health**
- **Providing opportunities to work and go back to school**

GET INVOLVED! Ask policy makers what they are doing about this issue. Look into what organizations that support marginalized youth are offering and how you can help. Watch the Homeless Hub for updates and more information.

SSHRC≡CRSH

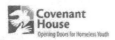

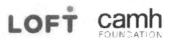

CHAPTER 6

Ethical Dilemmas in the Field: Reflections on Doing Research

This chapter continues from the previous chapters in terms of reflecting once again on the process of our work, in this case, the messiness of doing research. We examine the ethical and practical issues our team of researchers and research assistants confronted when conducting a longitudinal, mixed-methods study with our youth participants. In carrying out interviews, the research team began to raise a series of issues, ranging from the mundane to the epistemological. The post-modern turn in research and scholarship has been with us for over twenty-five years at this point, and has resulted in a more critical lens to bear on issues such as power, voice, representation, and interpretation and, as such, a general rethinking of the purposes and accounts that research can claim over its subjects. This chapter picks up on this discourse by examining "research as construct" (Lincoln & Cannella, 2009), interrogating the static notion of "Research" as an objective instrument of social scientific inquiry. We explore the nuances of researcher/researched relationships that arise in fieldwork; describe the "edges" and ethics of close relationships with participants; examine the complex issues that arise when monetizing research participation; and explore the ethics of ending relationships with research participants.

As the book's introduction notes, the study underpinning this chapter required research assistants to interview street youth four separate times over a one-year period. This longitudinal approach provides a unique contribution to the existing literature involving this population, which has generally captured experiences at a single point in time. In retrospect, the scale and depth of the study also provided an opportune chance to explore the epistemological and ethical challenges of conducting this research with a highly marginalized population, raising a host of serious issues to be considered by those conducting such research. This chapter argues that research of this kind must confront and work through a different kind of social science involving "not only a code of good conduct but a way of being that involves every aspect of one's soul" (Davidson, 1997, p. 123). In this way, we argue that working with populations such as homeless youth, particularly over time, demands confronting the limits of research, and that doing so provides researchers with a much more emancipatory opportunity to recast their research work as both a (modest) form of social justice and an ethical undertaking.

REFRAMING RESEARCH AND CONFRONTING THE LIMITS OF ETHICS

The work explored here has been a collective undertaking by a team of research assistants, project coordinators, and the four primary investigators of the study. The issues we encountered as a group were new to some, and were experienced in different contexts by more experienced members of the research team. Of course, in fields such as anthropology, ethical issues that arise from deeply engaging and forging relationships with study participants are hardly new, and have been grappled with extensively with no concrete resolution. As Richardson and McMullan (2007) argue, "nobody involved in researching 'the social' can avoid confronting ethical issues" (p. 115).

During data collection in both of our research sites, a host of methodological issues emerged that the team needed to deal with. For example, the research team began to note that the interviews were not a strict interaction between researcher and participant, but rather began to take on a relationship element since the researchers conducted four interviews with individual participants over a one-year period. This required a great deal of contact prior to the interview, often using text messaging as a mechanism for communication, to check in and determine a good time to conduct the interview, and gain (informal) consent to continue. The use of personal technology allowing one to instantly and informally connect with research participants is, of course, a new wrinkle in the process of becoming immersed in the field.

Many of the researchers involved in the project also came from a health promotion educational and training background, and reported feeling very "challenged" with "only collecting stories and information about people," without a formal mandate to intervene or engage participants in the realities of their situation. Recall that these youth were just getting off the street, and often expressed needs and problems that members of the research team were trained to help them with; but of course, in the context of the study, researchers were not ethically permitted to engage with participants as health professionals. In this way, the boundaries between researcher and participant felt "fuzzy" and "conflicting" to the research team. At the same time, the group wrestled with the longitudinal nature of the study. Many team members felt that, despite their attempts at maintaining a professional distance, they were undoubtedly becoming tied to research participants' lives and decision making. In effect, they were intervening despite the veneer of objectivity in the data collection. For instance, here is a simple exchange between participant and interviewer that neatly sums up the seemingly mundane manner in which this veneer began to subtly crack:

> **P:** Pretty bummed. 'Cause, I mean, I planned on moving but I wasn't sure, and I told them that. And they were like, "Well, if you need time, you know, take your time or whatever." But now, if I can't find a place or end up having a hard trouble with it then, yeah, I got to find somewhere to go whether I have someplace to go or not.
>
> **I:** Are they helping you find a place?
>
> **P:** No.
>
> **I:** Well, I don't know if you've ever heard about some of the programs. They have a housing worker who could help you, and she knows different landlords who are understanding of different situations. I can give you her name if you want to call her. I'm sure she might help out. She's helped other people.

P: Yeah, I would like that.

I: If you do want to get a place for then she might be able to hook you up. I don't know if it will be for March first. Her name's [Christy]. So I'll give you her information after.

P: Okay.

In this case—the second of four interviews—the nuanced entanglement of participant and interviewer comes into view. The exchange is simple, yet it raises a host of ethical questions about carrying out research with a vulnerable population. Accordingly, in this chapter we challenge our own assumptions, orientations, and experiences with the methodology employed, including the ethical issues that the study, once under way, presented to the research team. Further, we interrogate, however modestly, what Stewart (1996) coined "academic essentialism," and the desire for "decontaminated meaning." As a team, we open ourselves up to explore the uncertain space of error and representation, "displacing the rigid discipline of 'subject' and object' that sets Us apart and leaves Them inert and without agency" (Stewart, 1996, p. 26). This flattening and blurring of roles requires a nuanced and ongoing ethical strategy. Ethics protocols are ill-equipped to advise on the complex interactional dynamics that can emerge. Based on our experiences, we argue that such research requires a grounded ethical process. This process takes ethical ambiguity as a starting point and actively searches for ethical dilemmas to be used in further refining the research ethics strategy, just as a researcher would do with emergent themes in a grounded methodological strategy.

THE ETHICS AND EDGES OF INTIMACY

Ferrell and Hamm (1998) conceptualize fieldwork as "edge work," arguing that marginalized or deviant settings force researchers to straddle divides between legality and illegality, discredit and legitimacy, and morality and debauchery. They also contend that complete immersion in the field is necessary, and that sharing in the "pleasures and dangers" of a setting provides a more accurate reading of the lived realities where "crime and deviance" occur (Van Maanen, 1988). Stories from participants are often difficult to hear, and include experiences of drug use, physical/sexual abuse, mental illness, and the intersecting disadvantages of young lives lived on the street. The notion of being on the edge aptly and evocatively describes the many emotions our researchers experienced in their interactions with the youth involved in this study.

We attempted to balance the integrity of the interview with the emotional work it takes to engage the participant: demonstrating empathy and filling in the gaps and silences of an interview, while trying to maintain an open, nonjudgmental humanness to the interaction. Negotiating the ethical dimensions of this edge, between research intimacies, was an issue the entire team grappled with during the study. The challenges of negotiating this emotional edge were particularly salient during the first interviews with participants. When we asked youth about their personal histories, they recounted heart-wrenching stories of abandonment, abuse, and neglect. One female participant broke down in tears while discussing how hurt she had been by her parents' rejection, and how all she wanted was their love and support. Another explained that while he was disdainful of sex work, he felt forced to do it in order to make ends meet.

In classic feminist literature, Oakley (1981) argues that attempts to maintain detachment and distance with research participants serve to perpetuate inequalities and unequal power dynamics between researcher and subject. In this line of thinking, inequalities rooted in positivist "objective" approaches, which are embedded with what Smith (1991) would call the systemic relations of ruling, are overcome as researchers embrace the critique that impartial inquiry is not only impossible but highly problematic since the discourse of science is historically patriarchal. Intimacy is therefore valued as a way to "flatten the power gradient" (Swartz, 2011), hence the call to researchers to have "no intimacy without reciprocity" (Oakley, 1981). The obvious question that springs to mind, and which our previous examples of edge work highlight, is what to do if the researcher does not wish to share in the intimacy being presented to him or her.

The use of multiple interviews in this project meant that we built a unique sense of closeness or emotional connectedness with many of the young research participants, as we became regular parts of one another's lives over the course of a year. With a couple of these respondents, in particular, the connection was such that it led the interviewers to wonder if they might have been friends with the participants under different circumstances. In the context of this kind of mutual respect and intimacy, it was more tempting to disclose personal details and to offer advice. In one example, a participant came to the interview preoccupied with relationship trouble, and, over the course of two hours, the interview became an intimate conversation about relationships—an exchange that was meaningful for both parties, but which challenges traditional interview boundaries. We agreed as a team that this unique situation required us to challenge the typical role of objective researcher and to embrace the emotional labour required to bridge the gap in intimacy created by the research context. The team reasoned that we were asking a great deal of our research participants in such situations, and it seemed only fitting that we matched this emotional commitment by engaging with participants as individuals and not just subjects. From time to time, this took the form of members of the research team sharing personal information, stories, and experiences with the youth we were interviewing. This was a reoccurring theme that guided our ethical practice throughout the project, but which created issues of its own, as this chapter attests to and documents.

Another example of the emotional work of interviewing—one that illustrates the tensions surrounding this approach to intimacy—is the struggle to know when to challenge or confront harmful or negative attitudes and beliefs, and when to keep quiet in order to maintain rapport. This is a particularly tricky issue because it involves competing priorities: the need to find a balance between a commitment to the research (i.e., to ensuring data collection continues) and a desire to honour intimacy and engage with research participants honestly and not just as subjects. In one example, a particularly aggressive and confrontational participant would repeatedly make degrading and harmful comments about women and ethnic minorities, casually talk about being violent towards the women in his life, and then often look to the researcher to share in the "joke." Across interviews, particularly when asked about the future, participants expressed negative and self-deprecating beliefs about themselves and their self-worth. In such circumstances, the risk of challenging these beliefs is that it will provoke or embarrass the respondents and perhaps push them to drop out of the study. At the same time, the interviewer is working to create some level of trust and forge a nonjudgmental relationship with the participant, particularly during the first or second contact. When such situations arise, the interviewer is confronted with the ethics of simply "laughing along," disagreeing, or remaining silent. In the absence of a formalized and purposeful grounded ethical strategy to help identify and actively engage with this dilemma, the researchers in the above examples tended to default to a strategy of gently confronting respondents in order to emphasize their embarrassment: attempting to show some level of disapproval while still maintaining rapport. But the ethical question remains: Is this enough and is it the best course of practice? In reflecting on this situation after the fact, and returning to the view that research with vulnerable youth should engage with participants as honestly as possible, the research team feels that it would have been better for the interviewers to express their disapproval more directly. It seems disingenuous and unethical to step away from the role of objective researcher in emotional moments because that feels more honest and humanizing, but to reinstate that more detached role in other moments just because it helps us feel more comfortable. In support of this strategy, Swartz (2011) finds that being straightforward and nonindulgent with youth research participants actually improves rapport by facilitating a more honest relationship, and by working to break down power barriers.

While the notion of "flattening the power gradient" is admirable, one irony of framing research in this way is that our researchers also began to be confronted with their own privilege, latently manifest in relation to the research participants. The youth in the study tended to share common backgrounds and features, including low socio-economic familial contexts, low educational success, and what sociologists might generally describe as a low degree of both human and social capital. Conversely, those conducting the interviews were collectively struck by their own, quite opposite, life-course trajectories, with high degrees of educational success, resources, and ambitions. So, somewhat ironically, while feminist, post-structuralist, and post-modernist positionings have opened up spaces to question methodologies and the meta-narratives of objective social science, at the same time, they also raise new ethical issues. As England (1994) succinctly asks, "In our rush to be more inclusive and conceptualize difference and diversity, might we be guilty of appropriating the voices of 'others?'[And] can we incorporate the voices of 'others' without colonizing them in a manner that reinforces patterns of domination?" (p. 80). Irwin (2006), for example, cites feelings of "in-authenticity" in some research relationships, noting that friendships and intimacy can be "falsely and easily manipulated to hide the true goal of the relationship: to obtain rich data" (p. 158). Moreover, context is also critical to consider. Our study is one of an already vulnerable population: street youth. The danger—ethically, morally, and methodologically—is to ignore or not raise these issues through our research, and risk committing ourselves to an academic "ventriloquism" of the Other:

> No need to hear your voice when I can talk about you better than you can speak about yourself ... only tell me about your pain. I want to hear your story. And then I will tell it back to you in a new way ... I am still the author, authority. I am still the colonizer. (hooks, 1990, p. 343)

MONETIZING RESEARCH RELATIONSHIPS

The tension between the interview as a formal and professional interaction, and the interview as an opportunity for personal connection and intimacy, is further complicated in terms of providing honorariums to respondents. What does it mean to pay participants for their story? How does that shade the process of establishing intimacy and connection? In our research, our ethics application and strategy, to a degree, assumed some form of intervention: we paid each participant forty dollars for their time and effort per interview (up to four interviews), as an ethical strategy in the research. The study also built in the concept of a youth advisory committee, who could provide a loose member-checking protocol, and be actively involved with researchers in deciding how and where to communicate the results of the study. Three youth were trained in different technologies as possible avenues to disseminate the study's findings, and were invited to share those findings at an initial community meeting. It is also worth noting that throughout the data collection process there was an ongoing, and often informal, negotiation and discussion taking place between community housing workers and the research assistants and principal investigator(s) with respect to the research team's role, and what they could offer to the participants they were interviewing. The "expertise" offered by the researchers was typically mundane, but included information on services, key local contacts, or simply where to find bargains for everyday items.

Interestingly, while the notion of giving back is cited as one ethical strategy in research (Swartz, 2011), others take such a notion to task. Jeffrey (2006), for example, argues that research that simply pays participants is, or can be, patronizing. He maintains that vulnerable populations such as the poor (we use this strictly as an economic term) should be extended the opportunity to discuss their lives without always having to be given something in return. Based on our research experiences, we strongly disagree with such an assessment. Our team felt some measure of satisfaction with being able to provide the youth in the study—many of whom were just barely getting by financially in their new housing arrangements—with some much-needed funds. Swartz (2011) comments that emancipatory research, by its nature, seeks to ask participants what they want from the research process and from researchers. Given the team's extensive experience in working with this population, we were more than confident that the monetary offer was well received and in no way found to be patronizing. Upon arriving at a youth's home and providing the money, one researcher noted that the young person stated, "Oh man, great, I couldn't remember if this was the forty-dollar study or the other fifteen-dollar study ... so glad it's the forty-dollar one!"

This quotation also speaks to the fact that the youth we met are often interviewed many times about their experiences, and are repeating stories they have told other researchers and service providers. In this sense, many of the youth we engaged in the project are savvy research participants (Karabanow, 2006), which in itself illustrates that the young people participating in such research projects are likely also confronting the complexities of intimacy created by these interviews—what does it mean to them to get paid for sharing intimate details of their lives with researchers? We suggest that surest way to know is to ask, and that researchers should speak candidly with their participants about what they hope to get from the project, and the meaning of the honorarium. Even in our own research, these important questions were left to be addressed through a formal consent process that discusses honorariums in the most perfunctory of ways. This dialogue should emphasize that the honorarium is not payment for an individual's story, but a modest appreciation for the individual's expertise and time.

The importance of the forty-dollar honorarium for some respondents raises another ethical dilemma, in that the money can be seen to encourage individuals to participate in research when they might not otherwise. As a research team we had to confront the reality that many of our participants were keenly aware of the money and would have been unlikely to get involved in the study if there was less of a financial incentive. The honorarium also played a significant role in retention as we had participants contacting us in advance of their scheduled interview because they were facing financial hardship and saw the forty-dollar honorarium as a means to make ends meet. Our view is that the risk of inducement needs to be considered against the overall risk posed by the research. In the case of our research, because the risk associated with the research is relatively low, we feel that the incentive being offered was not such that it would encourage a potential respondent to assume a substantial amount of risk.

THE MESSINESS OF FIELDWORK

England (1994) aptly notes that in carrying out research "the field" is constantly changing; therefore, researchers must be able to manoeuvre around unexpected circumstances:

> The result is research where the only inevitability seems to be unreliability and unpredictability. This, in turn, ignites the need for a broader, less rigid conception of the "appropriate" method that allows the researcher flexibility to be more open to the challenges of fieldwork. (p. 81)

This is an appropriate summation of our team's experience, yet even such a comforting orientation to the uncertainness of research leaves one to grapple with the reality of carrying out research as a team in the field. For instance, our own researchers were uncertain how to navigate the gap between the formalized, bureaucratic details of the approved Research Ethics Board (REB) document and the actual circumstances they confronted, for example when the researcher did not believe the interviewee.

Indeed, for a group for whom standardized and legalized forms can carry connotations of justice and juvenile care systems, we often wondered if this medium (which seems to get longer and more complicated with every passing year) can actually deliver fully informed consent from marginalized people.

These ethical gaps raise a host of questions about the ethics of research and the evolution of research governance, from a system underpinned by the assumption of professional competence, to one largely designed to manage risks (Haggerty, 2004). For example, the Tri Council guidelines dictate that research participants must not be subjected to unnecessary risks or harm. As Haggerty (2004) points out, risk "has a precise meaning, most commonly associated with actuarial science where statistics about previous events are used to analyze the likelihood of future untoward potentialities" (p. 402).

In our study, the risks presented are often from the youth themselves, and the researchers are placed in a situation where they come to see or recognize a potential harm that is not rooted in empirical protocols, but rather is based on a feeling or statement that participants make about themselves or their situation. Identifying these harms is most definitely ad hoc and subjective, and ethics protocols do not typically provide guidelines for engaging with harms that emerge in the research process, but that are not specifically related to the research methodology. This underscores the need for a more grounded ethical strategy that is considerate of issues that fall outside standard ethics protocols. How do researchers address such harms when the act of intervening threatens the standards of objectivity and detachment? This dilemma is particularly pronounced in our study given our interest in studying life trajectories: by intervening, we potentially change the object of study (a young person's exit from homelessness).

Given the realities faced by our participants, our research team could not help but frame the data collection process as a form of intervention, regardless of whether or not the researcher explicitly "helped" or assisted the participant. Far removed (in the field) from the formal bureaucratic discourse of consent, harm, and risk, the researchers were required to make instant decisions about how to best support or help the person in front of them. Sometimes that meant saying nothing, sometimes it meant uncomfortably laughing along with crude or violent statements, and other times it required directing the person to a resource or service provider for help. As Haggerty (2004) concludes, "this is not to say that harms imagined by REBs are fictional, but that decisions about future potentialities are much more subjective and ad hoc than one might have concluded from the discourse of 'risk' used in the *Policy*" (p. 403).

RECIPROCITY AND DISTANCE

The requirement for informed consent in research is one of the central tenets of modern ethics, requiring that consent be voluntary, informed, and understood by the research subject. While the Tri-Council governing body in Canada requires one to explicitly sign a release acknowledging consent, and any risks that might entail, our team consistently struggled with what this acknowledgement permitted on our behalf (as research-ers and personal interlocutors). Intellectually, the notion of consent is simple to understand, explain, and document. In practice, it is complex, nuanced, and dynamic.

In the field with street youth, relationships and the "work" of ethics and consent become much more difficult to manage. As Renold, Holland, Ross, and Hillman (2008) note, "when the production of knowledge is collaboratively generated over time using participatory ethnographic methods (i.e. when purpose, aims, method and representation are up for negotiation) the ethics of how we come to 'know' and 'know well' are par-ticularly complex" (p. 434). For example, with respect to informed con-sent, how would youth, in reality, ever be able to fully consider consent through the longitudinal features of the research process they willingly consented to?

A particular instance of this complexity came into focus upon con-sideration of how the team would script the final interview. The youth shared intensely personal stories with the research team across the four interviews, and a tension began to arise between the ethical imperative to reciprocate those experiences and the practical task of ending data col-lection and therefore saying goodbye to the participant. England (1994) contends that, in general, relationships between the researcher and those being researched "may be reciprocal, asymmetrical, or potentially exploitive; and the researcher can adopt a stance of intimidation, ingratiation, self-promotion, or supplication" (p. 82). Our team chose a stance of supplication, meaning that as much as possible we acknowledged our reliance on the research subject, and employed methodological strategies that could assist us in dealing with asymmetrical and potentially exploitive power relations by explicitly acknowledging and confronting the limits of the research with our participants. Whether or not the participants did, or could, consent to our approach is, frankly, outside the purview of formal REB processes. To this end, the team decided to depart from the original interview script and developed a set of questions used during the final interview, which provided an opportunity for participants to speak to the power differentials inherent in the research process. This decision resulted from team meetings, and talking openly about the ethical and personal issues involved in conducting, and concluding, the research with participants. Here is an example of how this exchange opened up, however modestly, an opportunity to reflect and interrogate the formal research process:

I: Okay, but here's an interesting question: How has it been being a part of this study?

P: Good. It helped me.

I: You can be totally honest.

P: I've liked it because it gives me a chance to, not so much reach out, but again tell a story maybe in a different way because a lot of people, through this study, probably have similar stories ... and maybe they went in a totally different direction than me, somewhat different direction, or maybe made it half the way I did in the direction, and then maybe they had stable housing and then for some reason it got ripped out from underneath them and how that affected them. So, it gives a different, a different statistic. Some are highs, some are lows; even though someone might have stable housing ... but what's going on the inside?

In this way, the participant saw participation in the research as an effective way to contribute to what he perceived as the broader objective of the research, by telling his story in a "different way."

In such instances, and there were many, we glean insight into the agency on the other side of the (research) table: that research participants are themselves thinking about the why and how of the stories they tell, and are willingly scripting them to varying ends, along with the researcher. "Research" and the formalized discourse of REBs present the researcher as an expert guided by the notion of "do no harm," and objectified in the language of collecting data. Yet in this instance we see that the interview process is possible only through the willing participation, and perhaps even agenda, of the interviewee. Witness this exchange between researcher and participant, when the same question as in the example above was posed:

> **I:** What's it been like to be part of this study and meeting up every three months?
>
> **P:** A little bit intimidating because you being somebody who's university educated and successful and me being somebody who isn't, who sort of screwed that up, every day I was …
>
> **I:** Like a power imbalance kind of?
>
> **P:** Well, I don't know, you were a bit of a reminder of where I could be or where I should be, just, yeah.

Here, the power relations tacit in the exchange instead come to the surface. While the "power gradient" may have flattened through our approach over the course of the four interviews, there is no hiding the fact that the process drips with complex issues around voice, representation, and power. The academic desire for "decontaminated meaning" (Stewart, 1996) becomes antagonized by the agency of the interviewee, as the rigidity of Us and Them—of object and subject—begins to break down.

> **I:** Did you feel like it was because of the way I acted or just like the nature of the situation?
>
> **P:** The nature of the situation and just what you are. You're a successful, well-educated woman, right? So, and I'm uneducated by comparison and not successful, but I would say that the way you were, your personality and

everything, was what broke down those feelings and allowed me to open up and be honest with you. So, yeah, it was a little bit intimidating at first, but getting to know you and developing that rapport caused a bit of change there and I was fine after that.

In both cases, the hegemony of typical youth trajectories comes into full view as the participants contend that they, in some way, "failed" compared to the interviewer in what they perceive as a broader script of education and success (and no doubt comportment and appearance). The very fact that the interviewer is there to capture and hear their story of "failure" vis-à-vis their status of (albeit former) homelessness attests to the veracity of the participant's statement of "where [they] should be." Again, this speaks to the latent agency inherent in the interview: the interviewees are well aware of why they are being interviewed, and willingly choose which elements of their experiences they want to articulate.

CONCLUSION

While there is a dearth of qualitative longitudinal research with vulnerable populations, our research points to complex, and unique, methodological and ethical issues inherent to this kind of research. Following a period of mutual and common reflection, our team contends that researchers must think through the ethical issues and limits they will confront, and the strategies they may need to employ in response once data collection commences. Our experience with team data collection was that the standard ethical protocols were poor guidelines for many of the situations that presented themselves in the field. With REB approval in hand, and an intimate and sophisticated knowledge of the consent process and ethical processes rehearsed and understood, the team was still overwhelmed and, at times, underprepared for the realities of intimately engaging street youth and the unfolding dynamics of navigating the objective stance of "Research" in the field. Through our research, we hope to frankly acknowledge the ethical gaps, limitations, transgressions, and emotions that arise during research and data collection, alongside our hope to, however modestly, "help" those "subjects" whose stories we tell. While these stories, no matter how much we might theorize otherwise, must eventually be objectified as data in our own transcription, analysis, and scholarly work, our attempt here is to shed methodological light on how the data get worked up, and to suggest the need for more transparent and accountable field research processes in this area. In all, the realities of complex field relationships must be approached flexibly, with some advance planning, and the "messiness" of fieldwork should not be erased from the final research accounts.

CHAPTER 7

Conclusions

Most policy-makers, researchers, service providers, and young people would agree that the core part of a successful transition away from homelessness is stable housing. The interviews confirmed this, with many young people talking about how housing was an essential foundation for building confidence, and moving towards goals like getting back into school, finding a good job, addressing addictions issues, getting healthy, or reconnecting with family.

But we also found that the process of exiting homelessness actually started long before youth found stable housing. It began with a traumatic event or personal turning point that inspired them to dedicate themselves to the difficult task of getting away from the street. Youth encountered so many barriers to exiting homelessness that success was possible only when they were extremely committed and focused—a commitment that can be hard to maintain without a lot of help and support. This raises important questions about what we can collectively do to make this process less difficult for motivated young people.

As such, while it is remarkable that these young people found their way off the street, maintaining housing was often very challenging. Around 25 percent of the young people we interviewed lost their accommodations during the year of the study, and many of those who remained housed always thought that they were on shaky ground. A significant portion of our research population had been "transitioning away from homelessness" for years, with the overall process being two steps forward, one step back (or sometimes even two or three steps back).

The main reasons that the youth we interviewed lost their housing involved the following:

1. Roommate issues such as roommates not paying their portion of the rent or conflict with one another. With limited housing choices, young people were often forced to live with people whom they did not know very well, or who might be involved with crime or drugs.
2. Controlling or exploitative landlords who would not adequately maintain the unit, or who would try to impose rules outside of the bounds of the province's tenancy laws (telling people not to shower so much, or when they could come and go from their own apartment).
3. Outstanding legal trouble from long ago that finally resulted in jail time. Even a short time behind bars could lead youth to lose their housing.
4. Trouble with affordability. Young people who were unable to find subsidized housing often struggled to make ends meet while paying market rent, particularly in Toronto's high-priced rental market.
5. Ongoing addictions or mental health problems. These were ongoing issues for a number of the youth we talked to.

One of the central issues that young people encountered was social isolation. Youth experienced this loneliness and isolation because the transition from homelessness usually involved cutting themselves off from old friends. Young people often also broke ties with service agencies like shelters or drop-ins in order to avoid street culture, friends, and street activities. This social isolation can trigger a relapse in drug or alcohol problems, or exacerbate mental health issues like depression, anxiety, or PTSD, which are common among this group.

Finding employment was also a fundamental issue. Youth unemployment rates have been over 17 percent in Ontario and Nova Scotia for the last few years, and this is a group who is at a particular disadvantage because of limited work experience and criminal records (often for minor crimes related to survival or drug use, or due to the overpolicing of poor and homeless populations). Unemployment hurt young people financially and led to feelings of hopelessness. As noted at the beginning of this book, these findings about the main barriers and issues cut across our two research sites and underline for us the widespread and systemic nature of the issues the young people in our sample were facing.

We should point out that our findings are not all doom and gloom. There were many inspiring stories of resilience, strength, and success. We found that those young people who managed to find stable housing and begin working towards their personal goals felt they had the unconditional support of a family member, caseworker, or stable friend or romantic partner. Sadly, many of the people we interviewed did not have such a person, and even those who did continued to struggle. We also found that supportive and subsidized housing had a very positive impact by providing support and lessoning the financial burden young people faced. This was particularly true when they had more flexible rules that allowed for bumps in the road.

In reflecting on the implications of our research for policy, we came to realize that many of our recommendations for improvements have been around for a long time. At the risk of repeating these well-worn messages, governments at all levels need to invest more resources to address homelessness and to implement programs and initiatives that support systems-level planning and service integration. In particular, policy changes and sustained funding needs to be directed towards increasing housing affordability, increasing income supports (particularly for individuals with disabilities), improving access to mental health and addictions services, and removing systemic barriers to employment (particularly through the better management of criminal record checks).

More specifically, the results of the study support recent calls within the housing sector for homelessness policy to pivot away from a focus on emergency services to more focus on prevention and stabilization, strategies that prevent or disrupt damaging and costly cycles of homelessness before they really begin (Culhane & Metraux, 2008; Gaetz, O'Grady, Buccieri, et al., 2013). Building on this general perspective, the main recommendations for changes to policy and services from the findings of our research are as follows:

1. There needs to be enhancement of ongoing supports for young people who are transitioning from homelessness. This means that housing first efforts must maintain the strong social service supports that are at the heart of current approaches to homelessness. There is strong evidence that delayed transitions are economically costly, and that investment in youth transitions will be largely recouped through long-term cost savings. Beyond the profound human costs and the risks of long-term marginalization, delayed transitions are associated with significant financial costs in terms of ongoing unemployment, use of social assistance, contact with the criminal justice system, and increased use of emergency health services.

2. Transitioning young people need improved access to caseworker support that does not disappear when they age out of the social service system for homeless young people at the age of twenty-five. When possible, supports for transitioning young people should be decoupled from crisis-focused services for currently street-involved youth.

3. Interventions and supports need to directly address the barriers created by homelessness, such as limited work experience, stigma, limited opportunities due to police records, and the ongoing impacts of trauma. Access to support also needs to be streamlined in order to capitalize on transition points and to maintain momentum. There was nothing more demoralizing to youth than making big changes in their lives only to have unexpected barriers prevent further progress. Young people can be supported in maintaining momentum in positive changes with improved access to

   a. affordable housing and support in navigating tenancy,
   b. psychological and trauma counselling,
   c. record suspensions (formerly pardons), and follow-through on policies that remove non-conviction records from police record checks,
   d. family counselling and reconciliation services,
   e. drug treatment programs,
   f. skills-building, apprenticeship, work, and education opportunities,

g. programs that foster social interaction and provide healthy entertainment and stress relief (e.g., access to sports, arts, and bike repair programs).

As noted, in the one-year period of study, most of our participants were not making substantial gains in achieving health and stability. Of the fifty-one participants, 25 percent experienced a loss of stable housing over the year, and for all participants pathways were protracted and complex, with significant challenges in securing employment and decent-quality housing, and in engagement with educational programs (Frederick et al., 2014). Over the year there was no significant improvement in community integration, measures of mental health and quality of life varied erratically, and feelings of hope significantly declined (Kidd et al., 2016). It was found that having a community support worker, living in a supported housing context, and having a hopeful perspective mitigated threats to housing stability (such as criminal justice involvement or lack of employment). Furthermore, it was found that the more protracted the process of transitioning out of homelessness, the greater the difficulty youth had in achieving a reasonable quality of life, and of engaging in non-homeless communities (Kidd et al., 2016). Developing a sense of purpose and meaning was found to be essential to this process: youth found that housing had been oversold in terms of benefits. Many struggled greatly as they experienced social isolation, complex trauma-related symptoms, poor physical health, and other challenges.

Our participants, as a particular segment of the youth population who have transitioned out of basic homelessness, continue to describe their current lives in terms of fragility and instability. But while housing does not, in itself, shape these young people's sense of stability, it can positively influence feelings of health, happiness, and physical security. There are numerous interrelated factors at play that allow participants to regain a sense of citizenship and belonging in mainstream society. The complex and nuanced pathways from "street" to "mainstream" are fraught with uncertainty and struggle. In our research population, this journey occurs during emerging adulthood: a stage involving numerous developmental struggles (regarding identity, instability, self-focus, and feeling in-between), but also an age filled with possibilities. Indeed, it was a time when many of our participants experienced, as Arnett et al. (2014) describe, a new-found potential for handling responsibility, and of skill development and self-understanding.

Our study findings reinforce the critical need for service provid-ers—regardless of their philosophy, mandate, or mission—to make their resources known, easily accessible, and navigable for youth during their transition. In addition, evidence shows the need for agencies and servi-ces to be specifically tailored to homeless youth, and to have care pro-viders trained to understand the developmental needs and histories of this particular population. This can be achieved primarily through tar-geted outreach and follow-up programs, and services with caring staff members, a nonjudgmental atmosphere, and flexible policies (Garrett et al., 2008). While evidence demonstrates the positive impact that tar-geted treatment offered through programs like drop-in centres can have for homeless youth, if youth homelessness is to be successfully addressed, policy, funding, and service provision need greater focus, collaboration, and support (Slesnick et al., 2008).

For policy-makers, we hope our findings can trigger renewed atten-tion to growing evidence that the existence of diverse housing options catering to young adults significantly facilitates successful street exiting. Previous research has also highlighted critical problems with current public policies directed towards vulnerable youth in transition: eligibility criteria that exclude youth from services that might benefit them; inad-equate funding for transition services; a lack of coordination between ser-vice systems; and inadequate training about young-adult developmental issues for service professionals (Osgood, Foster, & Courtney, 2010). Clearly, what is needed is a developmentally appropriate and socially inclusive system of support for vulnerable youth as they move through adolescence into emerging adulthood.

Our study findings identified a critical need for change in services and policy. It also examined some creative art strategies to mobilize these findings—strategies not often considered by researchers. Indeed, we often fail to consider one of the greatest strengths offered by artwork, that of providing a common language to ensure end-user understand-ing. In order to begin to understand its full potential, art-focused know-ledge translation approaches deserve more exploration in future research, particularly regarding areas, such as homelessness, that are often marginalized and easily treated as siloes or overlooked by policy and practice sectors. For all of us, understanding the resilience and struggles of this population can provide compassion, empathy, and hope that it is possible to escape homelessness and take action to build healthier lives.

REFERENCES

Altena, A. M., Brilleslijper, S. N., & Wolf, J. L. M. (2010, June). Effective interventions for homeless youth: A systematic review. *American Journal of Preventive Medicine, 38*(6), 637–645. doi:10.1016/j.amepre.2010.02.017

Arnett, J. J., Žukauskienė, R., & Sugimura, K. (2014, December). The new life stage of emerging adulthood at ages 18–29 years: Implications for mental health." *Lancet Psychiatry, 1*(7), (569–576. doi:10.1016/S2215-0366(14)00080-7

Auerswald, C. L., & Eyre, S. L. (2002, May). Youth homelessness in San Francisco: A life cycle approach. *Social Science & Medicine, 54*(10), 1497–1512.

Baer, J. S., Peterson, P. L., & Wells, E. A. (2004, August). Rationale and design of a brief substance use intervention for homeless adolescents. *Addiction Research & Theory, 12*(4), 317–334.

Bannister, J., & O'Sullivan, A. (2013, November). Knowledge mobilisation and the civic academy: The nature of evidence, the roles of narrative and the potential of contribution analysis. *Contemporary Social Science, 8*(3), 249–262.

Barber, C. C., Fonagy, P., Fultz, J., Simulinas, M. A., & Yates, M. (2005, July). Homeless near a thousand homes: Outcomes of homeless youth in a crisis shelter. *American Journal of Orthopsychiatry, 75*(3), 347–355.

Baumstarck, K., Boyer, L., & Auquier, P. (2015, October). The role of stable housing as a determinant of poverty-related quality of life in vulnerable individuals. *International Journal of Quality in Health Care, 27*(5), 356–360. doi:10.1093/intqhc/mzv052

Boyatzis, R. E. (1998). *Transforming qualitative information: Thematic analysis and code development*. Thousand Oaks, CA: Sage.

Boydell, K. M., Goering, P., & Morrell-Bellai, T. L. (2000, January). Narratives of identity: Re-presentation of self in people who are homeless. *Qualitative Health Research, 10*(1), 26–38. doi:10.1177/104973200129118228

Brady, C., Moss, H., & Kelly, B. D. (2017). A fuller picture: Evaluating an art therapy programme in a multidisciplinary mental health service. *Medical Humanities, 43*(1), 30–34. doi:10.1136/medhum-2016-011040

Bronson, M. B. (2000). *Self-regulation in early childhood: Nature and nurture.* New York, NY: Guilford Press.

Buchko, A. A., Buchko, K. J., & Meyer, J. M. (2012, March). Is there power in PowerPoint? A field test of the efficacy of PowerPoint on memory and recall of religious sermons. *Computers in Human Behavior, 28*(2), 688–695.

Campbell-Grossman, C., Brage Hudson, D., Keating-Lefler, R., & Ofe Fleck, M. (2005, December). Community leaders' perceptions of single, low-income mothers' needs and concerns for social support. *Journal of Community Health Nursing, 22*(4), 241–257.

Campbell-Grossman, C. K., Hudson, D. B., Keating-Lefler, R., & Heusinkvelt, S. (2009, May). New mothers network: The provision of social support to single, low-income, African American mothers via e-mail messages. *Journal of Family Nursing, 15*(2), 220–236.

Clausen, J. A. (1998). Life reviews and life stories. In J. Z. Giele & G. H. Elder Jr. (Eds.), *Methods of life course research: Qualitative and quantitative approaches* (pp. 189–212). Thousand Oaks, CA: Sage.

Conrad, D. (2004). Exploring risky youth experiences: Popular theatre as a participatory, performative research method. *International Journal of Qualitative Methods, 3*(1), 12–25.

Cook, A., Spinazzola, J., Ford, J., Lanktree, C., Blaustein, M., Cloitre, M., ... van der Kolk, B. (2005, May). Complex trauma in children and adolescents. *Psychiatric Annals, 35*(5), 390–398.

Cornwall, A., & Jewkes, R. (1995, January). What is participatory research? *Social Science & Medicine, 41*(12), 1667–1676.

Coward Bucher, C. E. (2008, June). Toward a needs-based typology of homeless youth. *Journal of Adolescent Health, 42*(6), 549–554.

Culhane, D. P., & Metraux, S. (2008, January). Rearranging the deck chairs or reallocating the lifeboats? Homelessness assistance and its alternatives. *Journal of the American Planning Association, 74*(1), 111–121.

Dang, M. T., & Miller, E. (2013, November). Characteristics of natural mentoring relationships from the perspectives of homeless youth.

Journal of Child and Adolescent Psychiatric Nursing, 26(4), 246–253. doi:10.1111/jcap.12038

David, D. H., Gelberg, L., & Suchman, N. E. (2012, January). Implications of homelessness for parenting young children: A preliminary review from a developmental attachment perspective. *Infant Mental Health Journal, 33*(1), 1–9.

Davidson, A. I. (1997). *Foucault and his interlocutors.* Chicago, IL: University of Chicago Press.

Dawson, A., & Jackson, D. (2013, April). The primary health care service experiences and needs of homeless youth: A narrative synthesis of current evidence. *Contemporary Nurse, 44*(1), 62–75. doi:10.5172/conu.2013.44.1.62

Edidin, J. P., Ganim, Z., Hunter, S. J., & Karnik, N. S. (2012, June). The mental and physical health of homeless youth: A literature review. *Child Psychiatry & Human Development, 43*(3), 354–375.

Elliott, A. S., & Canadian Paediatric Society, Adolescent Health Committee. (2013, June). Meeting the health care needs of street-involved youth. *Paediatrics & Child Health, 18*(6), 317–326.

England, K. V. L. (1994, February). Getting personal: Reflexivity, positionality, and feminist research. *The Professional Geographer, 46*(1), 80–89.

Evenson, J., & Barr, C. (2009). *Youth homelessness in Canada: The road to solutions.* Toronto, ON: Raising the Roof.

Farrar, L., Schwartz, S. L., & Austin, M. J. (2011, March). Larkin Street Youth Services: Helping kids get off the street for good (1982–2007). *Journal of Evidence-Based Social Work, 8*(1–2), 106–123. doi:10.1080/15433714.2011.541826

Ferrell, J., & Hamm, M. S. (1998). *Ethnography at the edge: Crime, deviance, and field research.* Boston, MA: Northeastern University Press.

Forchuk, C., Ward-Griffin, C., Csiernik, R., & Turner, K. (2006, April). Surviving the tornado of mental illness: Psychiatric survivors' experiences of getting, losing, and keeping housing. *Psychiatric Services, 57*(4), 558–562.

Fortin, R., Jackson, S. F., Maher, J., & Moravac, C. (2015, March). I WAS HERE: Young mothers who have experienced homelessness use Photovoice and participatory qualitative analysis to demonstrate strengths and assets. *Global Health Promotion, 22*(1), 8–20. doi:10.1177/1757975914528960

Frederick, T. J., Chwalek, M., Hughes, J., Karabanow, J., & Kidd, S. (2014, November). How stable is stable? Defining and measuring housing stability. *Journal of Community Psychology, 42*(8), 964–979.

Gaetz, S., O'Grady, B., Buccieri, K., Karabanow, J., & Marsolais, A. (2013). *Youth homelessness in Canada: Implications for policy and practice.* Toronto, ON: Canadian Homelessness Research Network Press.

Gaetz, S., O'Grady, B., Kidd, S., & Schwan, K. (2016). *Without a home: The National Youth Homelessness Survey.* Toronto, ON: Canadian Observatory on Homelessness Press.

Gaetz, S., Scott, F., & Gulliver, T. (2013). *Housing First in Canada: Supporting communities to end homelessness.* Toronto, ON: Canadian Homelessness Research Network Press.

Gaetz, S. A., Donaldson, J., Richter, T., & Gulliver, T. (2013). *The state of homelessness in Canada—2013.* Toronto, ON: Canadian Observatory on Homelessness Press.

Garrett, S. B., Higa, D. H., Phares, M. M., Peterson, P. L., Wells, E. A., & Baer, J. S. (2008, November). Homeless youths' perceptions of services and transitions to stable housing. *Evaluation and Program Planning, 31*(4), 436–444.

Gassman, J., &. Gleason, M. C. (2011, January). The importance of mentoring relationships among youth workers. *New Directions for Youth Development, 2011*(S1), 55–76. doi:10.1002/yd.419

Goleman, D. (2006). *Emotional intelligence.* New York, NY: Bantam Books.

Gültekin, L., Brush, B. L., Baiardi, J. M., Kirk, K., & VanMaldeghem, K. (2014, November). Voices from the street: Exploring the realities of family homelessness. *Journal of Family Nursing, 20*(4), 390–414. doi:10.1177/1074840714548943

Hagan, J., & McCarthy, B. (1997). *Mean streets: Youth crime and homelessness.* Cambridge, UK: Cambridge University Press.

Haggerty, K. D. (2004, December). Ethics creep: Governing social science research in the name of ethics. *Qualitative Sociology, 27*(4), 391–414.

Head, B. W. (2008). Wicked problems in public policy. *Public Policy, 3*(2), 101–118.

Heath, C., & Heath, D. (2008). *Made to stick: Why some ideas survive and others die.* New York, NY: Random House.

Herrera, E., Jones, G. A., & Thomas de Benitez, S. (2009, February). Bodies on the line: Identity markers among Mexican street youth. *Children's Geographies, 7*(1), 67–81.

Holtrop, K., McNeil, S., & McWey, L. M. (2015, April). "It's a struggle but I can do it. I'm doing it for me and my kids": The psychosocial characteristics and life experiences of at-risk homeless parents in transitional housing. *Journal of Marital and Family Therapy, 41*(2), 177–191. doi:10.1111/jmft.12050

hooks, B. (1990). Marginality as a site of resistance. In R. Ferguson, M. Gever, T. T. Minh-ha, & C. West (Eds.), *Out there: Marginalization and contemporary cultures* (pp. 341–343). Cambridge, MA: MIT Press.

Housing first principles. (2017). Retrieved from The Homeless Hub website: http://homelesshub.ca/gallery/housing-first-principles

Hudson, A. L., Nyamathi, A., & Sweat, J. (2008, December). Homeless youths' interpersonal perspectives of health care providers. *Issues in Mental Health Nursing, 29*(12), 1277–1289. doi:10.1080/01612840802498235

Hughes, J. R., Clark, S. E., Wood, W., Cakmak, S., Cox, A., MacInnis, M., … Broom, B. (2010, November): Youth homelessness: The relationships among mental health, hope, and service satisfaction. *Journal of the Canadian Academy of Child & Adolescent Psychiatry, 19*(4), 274–283.

Irwin, K. (2006, June). Into the dark heart of ethnography: The lived ethics and inequality of intimate field relationships. *Qualitative Sociology, 29*(2), 155–175.

Jeffrey, R. (2006). Ethnography with the poor. Retrieved from http://www.educ.cam.ac.uk/RECOUP/documents/metpapers.pdf

Jenson, J. (2000). *Backgrounder: Thinking about marginalization: What, who and why?* Ottawa, ON: Canadian Policy Research Networks. Retrieved from http://cprn3.library.carleton.ca/documents/15746_en.pdf

Johnson, J. M. (2002). In-depth interviewing. In J. F. Gubrium & J. A. Holstein (Eds.), *Handbook of interview research: Context and method* (pp. 103–119). Thousand Oaks, CA: Sage.

Karabanow, J. (1999, October). Creating community: A case study of a Montreal street kid agency. *Community Development Journal, 34*(4), 318–327.

Karabanow, J. (2003, July). Creating a culture of hope: Lessons from street children agencies in Canada and Guatemala. *International Social Work, 46*(3), 369–386.

Karabanow, J. (2004a). *Being young and homeless: Understanding how youth enter and exit street life.* New York, NY: Peter Lang.

Karabanow, J. (2004b). *Exploring salient issues of youth homelessness in Halifax, Nova Scotia.* Ottawa, ON: Human Resources Development Canada Supportive Communities Partnership Initiative.

Karabanow, J. (2006). Becoming a street kid: Exploring the stages of street life. *Journal of Human Behavior in the Social Environment, 13*(2), 49–72.

Karabanow, J. (2008). Getting off the street: Exploring the processes of young people's street exits. *American Behavioral Scientist, 51*(6), 772–788.

Karabanow, J., Clement, P., Carson, A., & Crane, K. (2005). *Getting off the street: Exploring strategies used by Canadian youth to exit street life.* Toronto, ON: National Homelessness Initiative, National Research Program.

Karabanow, J., Hopkins, S., Kisely, S., Parker, J., Hughes, J., Gahagan, J., & Campbell, L. A. (2007, Summer). Can you be healthy on the street? Exploring the health experiences of Halifax street youth. *Canadian Journal of Urban Research, 16*(1), 12–32.

Karabanow, J., & Hughes, J. (2013). Building community: Supportive housing for young mothers. In S. Gaetz, B. O'Grady, K. Buccieri, J. Karabanow, & A. Marsolais (Eds.), *Youth homelessness in Canada: Implications for policy and practice* (pp. 111–130). Toronto, ON: Canadian Homelessness Research Network Press.

Karabanow, J., Hughes, J., Ticknor, J., Kidd, S., & Patterson, D. (2009). *Working within formal and informal economies: How homeless youth survive in neo-liberal times.* Ottawa, ON: Human Resources and Skills Development Canada.

Karabanow, J., Hughes, J., Ticknor, J., Kidd, S., & Patterson, D. (2010, December). The economics of being young and poor: How homeless youth survive in neo-liberal times. *Journal of Sociology and Social Welfare, 37*(4), 39–63.

Karabanow, J., & Naylor, T. (2015, December). Using art to tell stories and build safe spaces: Transforming academic research into action. *Canadian Journal of Community Mental Health, 34*(3), 67–85.

Kidd, S. A. (2003, August). Street youth: Coping and interventions. *Child and Adolescent Social Work Journal, 20*(4), 235–261.

Kidd, S. A. (2004, September). "The walls were closing in, and we were trapped": A qualitative analysis of street youth suicide. *Youth and Society, 36*(1), 30–55.

Kidd, S. A. (2006, June). Factors precipitating suicidality among homeless youth: A quantitative follow-up. *Youth and Society, 37*(4), 393–422.

Kidd, S. A. (2009, April). "A lot of us look at life differently": Homeless youths and art on the outside. *Cultural Studies <—> Critical Methodologies, 9*(2), 345–367.

Kidd, S. A. (2012, May). Seeking a coherent strategy in our response to homeless and street-involved youth: A historical review and suggested future directions. *Journal of Youth and Adolescence, 41*(5), 533–543.

Kidd, S. A. (2013). Mental health and youth homelessness: A critical review. In S. Gaetz, B. O'Grady, K. Buccieri, J. Karabanow, & A. Marsolais (Eds.), *Youth homelessness in Canada: Implications for policy and practice* (pp. 217–227). Toronto, ON: Canadian Homelessness Research Network.

Kidd, S. A., & Davidson. L. (2007, March). "You have to adapt because you have no other choice": The stories of strength and resilience of 208 homeless youth in New York City and Toronto. *Journal of Community Psychology, 35*(2), 219–238.

Kidd, S. A., Frederick, T., Karabanow, J., Hughes, J., Naylor, T., & Barbic, S. (2016, June). A mixed methods study of recently homeless youth efforts to sustain housing and stability. *Child and Adolescent Social Work Journal, 33*(3), 207–218.

Kidd, S. A., & Scrimenti, K. (2004, August). Evaluating child and youth homelessness: The example of New Haven, Connecticut. *Evaluation Review, 28*(4), 325–341.

Kidd, S. A., & Taub, B. G. (2004, July). A history of psychological research into the runaway phenomenon: From delinquent to street kid. *Journal of Social Distress and the Homeless, 13*(3–4), 327–343.

Kozloff, N., Adair, C. E., Palma Lazgare, L. I., Poremski, D., Cheung, A. H., Sandu, R., & Stergiopoulos, V. (2016, October). "Housing first" for homeless youth with mental illness. *Pediatrics, 138*(4), e20161514.

Lincoln, Y. S., & Cannella, G. A. (2009, April). Ethics and the broader rethinking/reconceptualization of research as construct. *Cultural Studies <—> Critical Methodologies, 9*(2), 273–285.

Mackelprang, J. L., Klest, B., Najmabadi, S. J., Valley-Gray, S., Gonzalez, E. A., & Cash, R. E. (2014, April). Betrayal trauma among homeless adults: Associations with revictimization, psychological well-being, and health. *Journal of Interpersonal Violence, 29*(6), 1028–1049. doi:10.1177/0886260513506060

Martijn, C., & Sharpe, L. (2006, January). Pathways to youth homelessness. *Social Science & Medicine, 62*(1), 1–12.

Mayberry, L. S. (2016, April). The hidden work of exiting homelessness: Challenges of housing service use and strategies of service recipients. *Journal of Community Psychology, 44*(3), 293–310.

Mayer, J. D., & Salovey, P. (1997). What is emotional intelligence? In P. Salovey & D. J. Sluyter (Eds.), *Emotional development and emotional intelligence: Educational implications* (pp. 3–31). New York, NY: Basic Books.

McKenzie-Mohr, S., Coates, J., & McLeod, H. (2012, January). Responding to the needs of youth who are homeless: Calling for politicized trauma-informed intervention. *Children and Youth Services Review, 34*(1), 136–143.

Milburn, N. G., Rice, E., Rotheram-Borus, M. J., Mallett, S., Rosenthal, D., Batterham, P., ... & Duan, N. (2009, December). Adolescents exiting homelessness over two years: The risk amplification and abatement model. *Journal of Research on Adolescence, 19*(4), 762–785.

Miller, W. L., & Crabtree, B. F. (2004). Depth interviewing. In S. Nagy Hesse-Biber & P. Leavy (Eds.), *Approaches to qualitative research: A reader on theory and practice* (pp. 185–202). New York, NY: Oxford University Press.

Nader-Grosbois, N. (2007). *Régulation, autorégulation, dysrégulation: Pistes pour l'intervention et la recherche.* Wavre, Belgium: *Éditions* Mardaga.

Narayan, A. J. (2015, March). Personal, dyadic, and contextual resilience in parents experiencing homelessness. *Clinical Psychology Review, 36*, 56–69. doi:10.1016/j.cpr.2015.01.005

Nelson, S. E., Gray, H. M., Maurice, I. R., & Shaffer, H. J. (2012, December). Moving ahead: Evaluation of a work-skills training program for homeless adults. *Community Mental Health Journal, 48*(6), 711–722.

Oakley, A. (1981). Interviewing women: A contradiction in terms. In H. Roberts (Ed.), *Doing feminist research* (pp. 30–61). London, UK: Routledge & Kegan Paul.

Ojeda, V. D., Hiller, S. P., Hurst, S., Jones, N., McMenamin, S., Burgdorf, J., & Gilmer, T. P. (2016, September). Implementation of age-specific services for transition-age youths in California. *Psychiatric Services, 67*(9), 970–976. doi:10.1176/appi.ps.201500084

Osei-Kofi, N. (2013, January). The emancipatory potential of arts-based research for social justice. *Equity & Excellence in Education, 46*(1), 135–149.

Osgood, D. W., Foster, E. M., & Courtney, M. E. (2010, Spring). Vulnerable populations and the transition to adulthood. *Future of Children, 20*(1), 209–229.

Perlman, S., Willard, J., Herbers, J. E., Cutuli, J. J., & Eyrich Garg, K. M. (2014, Fall). Youth homelessness: Prevalence and mental health correlates. *Journal of the Society for Social Work and Research, 5*(3), 361–377.

Peterson, P. L., Baer, J. S., Wells, E. A., Ginzler, J. A., & Garrett, S. B. (2006, September). Short-term effects of a brief motivational intervention to reduce alcohol and drug risk among homeless adolescents. *Psychology of Addictive Behaviors, 20*(3), 254–264.

Public Health Agency of Canada. (2006). *Street youth in Canada: Findings from enhanced surveillance of Canadian street youth, 1999–2003*. Ottawa, ON: Public Health Agency of Canada.

Quirouette, M., Frederick, T., Hughes, J., Karabanow, J., & Kidd, S. (2016, December). "Conflict with the law": Regulation and homeless youth trajectories toward stability. *Canadian Journal of Law and Society / La Revue Canadienne Droit et Société, 31*(3), 383–404.

Reason, P. (1998). Three approaches to participative inquiry. In N. K. Denzin & Y. S. Lincoln (Eds.), *Handbook of qualitative research* (pp. 324–339). Thousand Oaks, CA: Sage.

Renold, E., Holland, S., Ross, N. J., & Hillman, A. (2008, December). "Becoming participant": Problematizing "informed consent" in participatory research with young people in care. *Qualitative Social Work, 7*(4), 427–447.

Rew, L., & Horner, S. D. (2003, April). Personal strengths of homeless adolescents living in a high-risk environment. *Advances in Nursing Science, 26*(2), 90–101.

Richardson, S., & McMullan, M. (2007, December). Research ethics in the UK: What can sociology learn from health? *Sociology, 41*(6), 1115–1132.

Rodrigues Coser, L., Tozer, K., Van Borek, N., Tzemis, D., Taylor, D., Saewyc, E., & Buxton, J. A. (2014, September). Finding a voice: Participatory research with street-involved youth in the youth injection prevention project. *Health Promotion Practice, 15*(5), 732–738. doi:10.1177/1524839914527294

Rosenthal, D., Rotheram-Borus, M. J., Batterham, P., Mallett, S., Rice, E., & Milburn, N. G. (2007, November). Housing stability over two years and HIV risk among newly homeless youth. *AIDS and Behavior, 11*(6), 831–841.

Roy, É., Haley, N., Boudreau, J.-F., Leclerc, P., & Boivin, J.-F. (2009, January). The challenge of understanding mortality changes among street youth. *Journal of Urban Health, 87*(1), 95–101.

Roy, É., Haley, N., Leclerc, P., Sochanski, B., Boudreau, J.-F., & Boivin, J.-F. (2004, August). Mortality in a cohort of street youth in Montreal. *JAMA, 292*(5), 569–574.

Roy, É., Robert, M., Fournier, L., Laverdière, É., Berbiche, D., & Boivin, J.-F. (2016, February). Predictors of residential stability among homeless young adults: A cohort study. *BMC Public Health, 16*(1), 1–8. doi:10.1186/s12889-016-2802-x

Roy, É., Robert, M., Fournier, L., Vaillancourt, É., Vandermeerschen, J., & Boivin, J.-F. (2014, October). Residential trajectories of street youth—The Montréal cohort study. *Journal of Urban Health, 91*(5), 1019–1031.

Schrag, A., & Schmidt-Tieszen, A. (2014, August). Social support networks of single young mothers. *Child and Adolescent Social Work Journal, 31*(4), 315–327. doi:10.1007/s10560-013-0324-2

Shaw, M., & Dorling, D. (1998, August). Mortality among street youth in the UK. *Lancet, 352*(9129), 743.

Simpson, R. (2008). MIT young adult development project. Retrieved from http://hrweb.mit.edu/worklife/youngadult/index.html

Slesnick, N., Bartle-Haring, S., Dashora, P., Kang, M. J., & Aukward, E. (2008, April). Predictors of homelessness among street living youth. *Journal of Youth and Adolescence, 37*(4), 465–474.

Slesnick, N., Dashora, P., Letcher, A., Erdem, G., & Serovich, J. (2009, July). A review of services and interventions for runaway and homeless youth: Moving forward. *Children and Youth Services Review, 31*(7), 732–742.

Slesnick, N., & Prestopnik, J. L. (2005, April). Ecologically based family therapy outcome with substance abusing runaway adolescents. *Journal of Adolescence, 28*(2), 277–298.

Slesnick, N., Prestopnik, J. L., Meyers, R. J., & Glassman, M. (2007, June). Treatment outcome for street-living, homeless youth. *Addictive Behaviors, 32*(6), 1237–1251.

Smith, D. (1991). *The rise of historical sociology*. Cambridge, UK: Polity Press.

Smith, R. (2010, September). Antislick to postslick: DIY books and youth culture then and now. *Journal of American Culture, 33*(3), 207–216.

Snyder, C. R., Harris, C., Anderson, J. R., Holleran, S. A., Irving, L. M., Sigmon, S. T., … Harney, P. (1991, April). The will and the ways: Development and validation of an individual-differences measure of hope. *Journal of Personality and Social Psychology, 60*(4), 570–585.

Star, K. L., & Cox, J. A. (2008, December). The use of phototherapy in couples and family counseling. *Journal of Creativity in Mental Health, 3*(4), 373–382.

Stergiopoulos, V., Gozdzik, A., O'Campo, P., Holtby, A. R., Jeyaratnam, J., & Tsemberis, S. (2014, April). Housing first: Exploring participants' early support needs. *BMC Health Services Research, 14*(1), 167. doi:10.1186/1472-6963-14-167

Stewart, K. (1996). *A space on the side of the road: Cultural poetics in an "other" America*. Princeton, NJ: Princeton University Press.

Swartz, S. (2011, February). "Going deep" and "giving back": Strategies for exceeding ethical expectations when researching amongst vulnerable youth. *Qualitative Research, 11*(1), 47–68.

Tesch, L., & Hansen, E. C. (2013, February). Evaluating effectiveness of arts and health programmes in primary health care: A descriptive review. *Arts & Health: An International Journal for Research, Policy and Practice,* 5(1), 19–38.

Tevendale, H. D., Comulada, W. S., & Lightfoot, M. A. (2011, December). Finding shelter: Two-year housing trajectories among homeless youth. *Journal of Adolescent Health, 49*(6), 615–620.

Tozer, K., Tzemis, D., Amlani, A., Coser, L., Taylor, D., Van Borek, N., … Buxton, J. A. (2015, August). Reorienting risk to resilience: Street-involved youth perspectives on preventing the transition to injection drug use. *BMC Public Health, 15*(1), 1–11.

United Nations Educational, Scientific and Cultural Organization. (2014). Street children. Retrieved from http://www.unesco.org/new/en/social-and-human-sciences/themes/fight-against-discrimination/education-of-children-in-need/street-children/

Urwyler, P., Rampa, L., Stucki, R., Büchler, M., Müri, R., Mosimann, U. P., & Nef, T. (2015, June). Recognition of activities of daily living in healthy subjects using two ad-hoc classifiers. *Biomedical Engineering Online, 14*(1), 54. doi:10.1186/s12938-015-0050-4

Van Maanen, J. (1988). *Tales of the field: On writing ethnography.* Chicago, IL: University of Chicago Press.

Walsh, D. (2008). Creative expressions: Art therapy in a community context. In A. Lewis & D. Doyle (Eds.), *Proving the practice: Evidencing the effects of community arts programs on mental health* (pp. 74–83). Fremantle, Australia: DADAA.

Wenzel, S., Holloway, I., Golinelli, D., Ewing, B., Bowman, R., & Tucker, J. (2012, May). Social networks of homeless youth in emerging adulthood. *Journal of Youth and Adolescence, 41*(5), 561–571. doi:10.1007/s10964-011-9709-8

White, M. (2006, May). Establishing common ground in community-based arts in health. *Journal of the Royal Society for the Promotion of Health, 126*(3), 128–133.

Windsor, J. (2005). *Your health and the arts: A study of the association between arts engagement and health.* London, UK: Arts Council England.

Wong, C. F., Clark, L., F., & Marlotte, L. (2016, March). The impact of specific and complex trauma on the mental health of homeless youth. *Journal of Interpersonal Violence, 31*(5), 831–854.

INDEX